COPING V

SHIRLEY TRICKETT
ing a counsellor and te.... ... ... is ue author of *The Irritable Bowel Syndrome and Diverticulosis* and *Coming off Tranquillisers and Sleeping Pills* (both published by Thorsons). Her other books include *Coping with Anxiety and Depression*, *Coping Successfully with Panic Attacks* and *Coping with Candida* (all Sheldon Press). In 1987 she won a Whitbread Community Care Award.

Overcoming Common Problems Series

For a full list of titles please contact
Sheldon Press, Marylebone Road, London NW1 4DU

Antioxidants
DR ROBERT YOUNGSON

The Assertiveness Workbook
A plan for busy women
JOANNA GUTMANN

Beating the Comfort Trap
DR WINDY DRYDEN AND JACK
GORDON

Birth Over Thirty Five
SHEILA KITZINGER

Body Language
How to read others' thoughts by their
gestures
ALLAN PEASE

Body Language in Relationships
DAVID COHEN

Calm Down
How to cope with frustration and anger
DR PAUL HAUCK

Cancer – A Family Affair
NEVILLE SHONE

The Candida Diet Book
KAREN BRODY

Caring for Your Elderly Parent
JULIA BURTON-JONES

Cider Vinegar
MARGARET HILLS

Comfort for Depression
JANET HORWOOD

Coping Successfully with Hayfever
DR ROBERT YOUNGSON

**Coping Successfully with Joint
Replacement**
DR TOM SMITH

Coping Successfully with Migraine
SUE DYSON

Coping Successfully with Pain
NEVILLE SHONE

Coping Successfully with Panic Attacks
SHIRLEY TRICKETT

Coping Successfully with PMS
KAREN EVENNETT

**Coping Successfully with Prostate
Problems**
ROSY REYNOLDS

**Coping Successfully with Your Hiatus
Hernia**
DR TOM SMITH

**Coping Successfully with Your Irritable
Bladder**
JENNIFER HUNT

**Coping Successfully with Your Irritable
Bowel**
ROSEMARY NICOL

Coping with Anxiety and Depression
SHIRLEY TRICKETT

Coping with Blushing
DR ROBERT EDELMANN

Coping with Breast Cancer
DR EADIE HEYDERMAN

Coping with Bronchitis and Emphysema
DR TOM SMITH

Coping with Candida
SHIRLEY TRICKETT

Coping with Chronic Fatigue
TRUDIE CHALDER

Coping with Coeliac Disease
KAREN BRODY

Coping with Cystitis
CAROLINE CLAYTON

Coping with Depression and Elation
DR PATRICK McKEON

Coping with Eczema
DR ROBERT YOUNGSON

Coping with Endometriosis
JO MEARS

Coping with Fibroids
MARY-CLAIRE MASON

Coping with Headaches
SHIRLEY TRICKETT

Coping with a Hernia
DR DAVID DELVIN

Coping with Psoriasis
PROFESSOR RONALD MARKS

Coping with Rheumatism and Arthritis
DR ROBERT YOUNGSON

Coping with Stammering
TRUDY STEWART AND JACKIE
TURNBULL

Coping with Stomach Ulcers
DR TOM SMITH

Coping with Strokes
DR TOM SMITH

Overcoming Common Problems Series

Coping with Thrush
CAROLINE CLAYTON

Coping with Thyroid Problems
DR JOAN GOMEZ

Coping with Your Cervical Smear
KAREN EVENNETT

Crunch Points for Couples
JULIA COLE

Curing Arthritis
More ways to a drug-free life
MARGARET HILLS

Curing Arthritis Diet Book
MARGARET HILLS

Curing Arthritis – The Drug-Free Way
MARGARET HILLS

Curing Arthritis Exercise Book
MARGARET HILLS AND JANET
HORWOOD

Cystic Fibrosis – A Family Affair
JANE CHUMBLEY

Depression
DR PAUL HAUCK

Divorce and Separation
Every woman's guide to a new life
ANGELA WILLANS

**Everything Parents Should Know About
Drugs**
SARAH LAWSON

Feverfew
DR STEWART JOHNSON

Gambling – A Family Affair
ANGELA WILLANS

Garlic
KAREN EVENNETT

The Good Stress Guide
MARY HARTLEY

Heart Attacks – Prevent and Survive
DR TOM SMITH

**Helping Children Cope with Attention
Deficit Disorder**
DR PATRICIA GILBERT

Helping Children Cope with Bullying
SARAH LAWSON

Helping Children Cope with Divorce
ROSEMARY WELLS

Helping Children Cope with Dyslexia
SALLY RAYMOND

Helping Children Cope with Grief
ROSEMARY WELLS

Helping Children Cope with Stammering
JACKIE TURNBULL AND TRUDY
STEWART

Hold Your Head Up High
DR PAUL HAUCK

How to Be Your Own Best Friend
DR PAUL HAUCK

How to Cope When the Going Gets Tough
DR WINDY DRYDEN AND JACK
GORDON

How to Cope with Anaemia
DR JOAN GOMEZ

How to Cope with Bulimia
DR JOAN GOMEZ

How to Cope with Difficult Parents
DR WINDY DRYDEN AND JACK
GORDON

How to Cope with Difficult People
ALAN HOUEL WITH CHRISTIAN
GODEFROY

**How to Cope with People who Drive You
Crazy**
DR PAUL HAUCK

How to Cope with Splitting Up
VERA PEIFFER

How to Cope with Stress
DR PETER TYRER

How to Enjoy Your Retirement
VICKY MAUD

How to Improve Your Confidence
DR KENNETH HAMBLY

How to Interview and Be Interviewed
MICHELE BROWN AND GYLES
BRANDRETH

How to Keep Your Cholesterol in Check
DR ROBERT POVEY

How to Love and Be Loved
DR PAUL HAUCK

How to Pass Your Driving Test
DONALD RIDLAND

How to Stand up for Yourself
DR PAUL HAUCK

**How to Start a Conversation and Make
Friends**
DON GABOR

How to Stick to a Diet
DEBORAH STEINBERG AND
DR WINDY DRYDEN

How to Stop Worrying
DR FRANK TALLIS

How to Succeed as a Single Parent
CAROLE BALDOCK

Overcoming Common Problems Series

Overcoming Common Problems

Coping with Headaches

Shirley Trickett

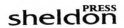
sheldon**PRESS**

First published in Great Britain in 1999 by
Sheldon Press, SPCK, Marylebone Road, London NW1 4DU

British Library Cataloguing-in-Publication Data
A catalogue record for this book is available from the British Library

ISBN 0–85969–812–2

Typeset by Deltatype Limited, Birkenhead, Merseyside
Printed in Great Britain by
Biddles Ltd, Guildford and King's Lynn

Contents

For my twin sister Sheila and her
husband Henricus, the love and support of whom
have saved me many a 'headache'

Introduction

In headaches and worry life leaks away

W. H. AUDEN

For the past 15 years I have worked with the public, teaching self-help methods for relief of all types of pain, sore heads, aching shoulders, backs tight with muscle spasm, the pain of drug addiction, the pain of loss and, perhaps hardest of all to witness, depression, the pain of loss of self. Pain hurts – it's meant to – it alerts us to the fact that something is wrong, that we must act.

Common headaches respond well to self-help methods and there are several avenues suggested in this book for you to explore to discover why you are having headaches. There are also many practical measures given for relieving your symptoms.

Working towards wholeness

Release from pain often brings the energy necessary for change. Is it time for you to stop 'beating yourself with sticks': I should do this, I should do that? Is it time for you to discover who you really are, to find your own truth and not be contented with the fake picture of self you have come to accept – a collage of impressions built up initially from feedback from parents/siblings/teachers and, in your adult life, from what your partner/boss/friends and others say you are?

Allowing yourself as long as it takes

Taking the time to discover what is causing your headaches could also be the time for taking a compassionate look at yourself and perhaps looking at 'the pain beyond the pain' – the suppressed aspects of self, your deep needs and desires – a time for retaining only the learning from past emotional pain and letting go of the rest.

Acceptance of who you are

Until you accept that you are a special being worthy of self-respect and love it is unlikely that you will find the inner peace necessary to work towards true health – the harmonious interaction of body, mind, emotions and spirit. As feelings of self-worth grow so will your confidence, and as old fears recede the crutches of addictions, obsessions, overdependence on relationships and work can be discarded, and as you love yourself and become centred in your being you can continue on your chosen path with a much lighter step.

'Love is the highest degree of medicine' – PARACELSUS

Shirley Trickett

1

The volcano effect

It is unlikely that your headache will have a single precipitating factor. Chronic headaches can be the end result of a long chain of events. You might have been laying the fundation stones for your headaches for many years, possibly since childhood, even since birth, with that first monumental headache that was necessary for your entry into the world.

The smouldering volcano

Think of your body as a volcano, a baseline of seismic activity. The smouldering comes from your physical, emotional and spiritual reactions to your life circumstances, which provide a continual background of strain. It then only needs a trigger for it to explode into a full-blown eruption – your headache.

What is the function of a headache?

Your body, far from letting you down when it produces a headache, is trying to make you aware of how harshly you are treating it, and it will continue to plague you with pain until you listen. It is trying to make you change some aspect, or possibly more than one destructive pattern of behaviour – trying to get you to stop and *think*.

A headache enforces rest

It might be saying to you: why do you continually overwork/when are you going to look to your emotional needs/when are you going to eat sensibly/when are you going to cut down on alcohol/when are you going to get out of that relationship/when are you going to realize your immune system is very low/when are you going to follow your life purpose? The list is endless.

Beginning at the beginning

Many people understandably become obsessed by the headache but fail to see it as an end result, not the start of their problems or how they are treating their body. 'If only I did not get these headaches

1

life would be wonderful.' This is unlikely; headaches don't evolve without favourable conditions and, in any case, if you did not get headaches nature might prod you in some other way to force you to take stock. It could be by giving you digestive problems, panic attacks, asthma, depression or any chronic condition which forces you temporarily to slow down. Which condition manifests in you will depend on where your weak spot is. Have you noticed that when a long-term stress-induced malady for some reason disappears *there is always another one standing in the queue ready to take its place*? Perhaps this is the body saying, 'Well if you won't listen to what a gastric ulcer is telling you let's try panic attacks – they can lead to agoraphobia and then see if you can carry on working at this pace!'

All recurrent conditions highlight the fact that your being is not balanced, is not in harmony. This is the baseline. This is where your detective work begins, taking an honest look at what is smouldering at the bottom of your volcano and being open enough to admit that whatever is lurking there is your responsibility, not your doctor's (providing, of course, that he has fully investigated your symptoms). Nor are they the fault of your boss/partner/mother-in-law. You cannot change their behaviour no matter how unreasonable it is. All you have control over is your reaction to your position – how much you are going to allow yourself to be affected and, in short, how much you are going to stoke the fires of your volcano.

But my headaches are purely physical

You might want to protest, 'But it is only stuffy rooms/sinus problems/sunlight/loud noise and so on that affects me. It is physical.' Nothing can be 'just physical' – the autonomic nervous system is governed by the emotions, which in turn affect the circulation, the muscles, the immune system and so on, and although this may be a bit esoteric for some, I believe that the emotions depend on the spirit. So everything affects everything else. If you find all this discouraging and wonder where to start, remember that the good news is, because of this interdependency, any positive actions towards balance in one area will affect the whole being.

2

List of suspects

This book aims to encourage headache sufferers to turn detective and discover what is causing their headaches. The holistic, active role is stressed and it is hoped that sufferers will be excited by the opportunity to participate in their own improved health or cure. Headaches are rarely fatal, but they can cause great distress, not only because they can be such agony but also because they can destroy self-esteem and the ability to cope. They can also be responsible for loss of employment and loss of relationships, and lead to suicidal depression.

The book describes different types of headaches, lists common causes and discusses a variety of simple self-help treatments. It presupposes that the reader's symptoms have been investigated by his/her doctor, that a firm diagnosis has been made and that the type of headache diagnosed falls into the group which responds well to self-help methods. This group includes tension headaches, migraine, allergic headaches and many more, as you will see when you read on.

What is a headache?

A headache is a pain in the head which can range from a slight ache that makes life a bit dreary, but does not seriously affect concentration, to a pain so disabling that the thought process is severely disturbed and the sufferer is completely prostrate. The degree of pain is usually determined by the amount of swelling in the soft tissue of the head. It is easy to see why this can be so agonizing: if your arm needed to swell it is free to do so, but since the brain is confined by the bony case of the skull there is no relief until the swelling subsides. Common descriptions of headaches suggest this pressure: 'I thought my head would split', 'I felt as though my head was in a vice.'

What is a headache saying?

A headache is the head saying that you are subjecting it to conditions it cannot tolerate. A mild headache may be saying, 'Can't you do something about this?'; a severe headache caused by poisonous fumes may be saying 'Get out of here, your life is in danger.'

Headaches don't descend on us without reason and you may have to accept that, however unwittingly, you are actually causing yours. This will become clearer as you understand the needs of the head:

- normal circulation
- nourishment
- the correct balance of oxygen and carbon dioxide
- absence of toxic substances.

In a healthy person it is unlikely that a headache would develop if these needs are met.

Common headaches

Tension	Caused by contraction of the muscles.
Migraine	Caused by altered circulation to the head.
Hormonal	Caused by changing hormone levels, for example, premenstrual tension, the menopause, taking the pill.
Post-stress	Caused by dilation of blood vessels after period of constriction.
Allergic	Caused by exposure to pollens, moulds, chemicals, foods.
Infective	Caused by bacteria or viruses.
Structural	Caused by bones being out of alignment, for example the jaw bone.
Postural	Caused by putting a strain on the muscles of the head, neck and shoulders.
Eye strain	Caused by overuse of the muscles around the eyes.
Hypoglycaemic	Caused by rapid changes in the blood sugar levels; dieting, poor nutrition, irregular meals.
Toxic	Caused by overindulgence in food and drink, constipation, absorption of toxins from the colon.
Drug-induced	Caused either by ingestion of drugs or as part of the withdrawal reaction.

4

Hyperventilation	Caused by an unbalanced mixture of oxygen and carbon dioxide in the brain.
Atmospheric	Caused by geopathic stress – gases, radiation, positive ions, stuffy rooms.
Electrical pollution	Caused by power cables, VDUs, etc.

Which type of headache?

There are two main types of headache and if you can decide which one plagues you, then the causes will be easier to pinpoint and it will be easier to find effective treatment.

Tight-muscle (tension) headaches

This is the most common type of headache. When muscles in the head, neck or shoulders are shortened (contracted), blood vessels are constricted and the circulation to the brain is affected. The neck is the gateway to the head and if this gate is partially closed the results are dull headaches, woolly thinking, dizziness and irritability. Many sufferers from this type of headache are unaware of the extent of the congestion in their muscles until firm pressure around the base of the skull, the back of the neck or the shoulders causes them to howl in protest. When the blood circulates freely the waste products of metabolism (the burning of the food we eat) are rinsed away and excreted. When the muscles are tight the waste products are trapped and form crystals. It is when these are pressed on to the bones that the pain is felt. If you are tender in these muscles and your headache is relieved by a head and shoulder massage, you can be fairly sure it is a *tight-muscle or tension headache*. Alcohol is a powerful muscle relaxant so if your symptoms are improved by a drink, this could confirm the diagnosis.

Appearance of person with tension headache

If the blood vessels are dilated the face can be flushed or puffy and the eyes bloodshot. If the blood vessels are contracted the face is usually pale. One or both shoulders can be pulled up towards the ears, the head can be inclined to one side or the chin may be jutting forward in the turtle position. Why this happens will be explained later. Lying flat can increase blood flow to the head and relieve symptoms. Muscular headaches can be caused by stress, trauma,

5

posture, allergies, infections, low body temperature and low blood sugar. Sometimes it is not just one factor but a combination that starts a headache.

Dilated-blood-vessel (vascular) headaches

The pain in this type of headache is usually caused by pressure on the nerves as the blood vessels swell. Migraine and hormonal headaches, such as those experienced premenstrually and during the menopause, could be in this group. Alcohol and lying flat, because they increase blood flow to the head, usually make the symptoms worse.

Appearance of person with vascular headache

If the blood vessels are dilated the face can be flushed or puffy and the eyes bloodshot. If the blood vessels are contracted the face is usually pale.

Combination headaches

You may get different types of headaches at different times or sometimes you may feel you have a mixture of the two types. The pain from a vascular headache can cause you to tighten head and neck muscles and so compound the problem.

It's your *head*

If your doctor has ruled out conditions which would cause headaches, such as high blood pressure, and you have recently had your eyes tested, it is really up to you to discover what you are doing in your daily routine to make your head object so strongly. Some people become angry when their doctor cannot reveal the cause of their headaches, and feel discouraged when they leave the surgery with yet another prescription for painkillers. They are often reluctant to take these, either because they don't find them very effective or because they feel they have been on drugs for too long. If you feel angry with your doctor, try to remember that he is probably not disputing that you have headaches, only that he is baffled by the cause. Don't be worried by the diagnosis 'ideopathic headaches'; this only means headaches of unknown origin. After you have read the next chapters (and always assuming that your doctor has ruled

6

out any serious disorder), you will see that it makes more sense for you to be the sleuth because he/she cannot know enough about your life to pinpoint one of the multitude of causes.

Tension and vascular headaches will be looked at in more detail in Chapters 4 and 5. The next chapter alerts you to some medical emergencies.

3

When to call the doctor:
Headaches which need urgent or continued medical attention

Medical instructions must be followed at all times. Do not cut down or stop medication or change your treatment in any way without consulting your doctor.

Having said that, there are many headaches where self-help methods enhance the conventional medical treatment. For example, if you have severe sinusitis and need an antibiotic, using steam inhalations or essential oils as well can reduce swelling and ease pain, and taking supplements which will stop the antibiotics upsetting your digestion or giving you thrush can only be of value. The other great benefit of self-help is learning what to do to prevent further attacks (prophylactic treatment). For example, if you understand that depleting your immune system is asking for repeated infections and you take steps to correct this, it could turn you from a passive prescription-taker to a person who has enough knowledge to avoid or limit further attacks.

When to seek medical help

After injury

Headaches after injury should always be investigated even if the onset is some time after the injury. This does not mean you need to rush off to the doctor every time your child bumps its head, but if the colour does not return to the face of the child (or adult), and there is vomiting, drowsiness, irritability or loss of consciousness, seek urgent help. It could be that there is increased pressure in the brain (intracranial) due to swelling or bleeding.

Any sudden severe headache

Unless the person is a known headache sufferer where the cause has been established and the symptoms are the same as in previous attacks, seek help. Known headache sufferers, say a person who has tension headaches or migraine, are not immune from other causes of severe headaches such as strokes.

Known headache sufferers

If the nature of the headache changes in frequency or severity, if the usual treatment affords no relief or if the pain is accompanied by any new symptoms, including:

- blackouts
- dizziness
- visual disturbances
- speech difficulties: either difficulty making the tongue work properly or inability to remember words
- clumsiness
- muscle weakness or numbness
- incontinence
- depression

seek help and explain any new symptoms to the doctor. He/she might want to review diagnosis and treatment.

Don't panic

If you have developed any symptoms which your doctor does not know about or any of the above symptoms, you should seek medical attention, but there is no need to panic and assume you have some serious illness. The same symptoms can be found in many conditions such as migraine, drug withdrawal and severe anxiety.

Prescribed drugs

If you have been given new medication for any condition and you develop headaches, consult your doctor. Headaches are a side-effect of many drugs and you may be told that they are to be expected and will ease off as your body adjusts to the drug. If, however, the headaches are severe and are accompanied by a rash or nausea, it could also be that you are having an allergic reaction. Prompt medical attention should be sought.

Headaches with fever

A headache can be expected with an infection such as flu and can usually be eased by a couple of aspirin or paracetamol. Seek help if:

- the pain is severe and the onset sudden

- there is vomiting
- neck stiffness
- a rash
- aversion to light
- high-pitched crying (children).

These symptoms appear in meningitis.

Headaches with fever, facial pain, earache or sore throat

Always seek medical help, especially in children. An antibiotic may be indicated.

Severe pain in the temple

Severe pain with swollen blood vessels in the temple region, sometimes with generalized muscle and joint pains: these symptoms appear in a condition called temporal arteritis (inflammation of the temporal arteries). This is a serious condition which needs urgent medical help. The middle-aged and elderly are most at risk of developing this but it is occasionally seen in younger people.

Headaches with eye pain or visual disturbances

Report all headaches with eye pain or visual disturbances to a doctor immediately. They do occur in migraine but can also be glaucoma, a serious disease of the eye which needs prompt treatment. The symptoms come from impaired drainage of the fluid from the eye. The pain can be severe or mild and is felt around one or both eyes, or in the forehead. Nausea and vomiting may be present. Many individuals suffering from glaucoma see coloured halos around lighted objects or experience mistiness of vision. Some drugs worsen this condition, including: antihistamines, some bowel relaxants, certain tranquillizers, the tricyclic antidepressants, some anti-sickness drugs, some drugs used in Parkinson's disease (Saper and Magee, 1978). Over-the-counter headache preparations should be avoided until you have seen your doctor.

While some symptoms have been highlighted in this chapter to alert you to medical emergencies, absence of these symptoms does not mean you do not need medical help. Always consult your doctor if you have headaches.

Is it a tumour?

This is the major anxiety of most new headache sufferers. Ninety-five per cent of the population have headaches at some time. Tumours as a cause of these are rare. Other symptoms of a tumour are likely to take you to the doctor before a headache does (Blau, 1991).

4

Muscular-contraction or tension headaches

Tension or muscular-contraction headaches probably affect more people than any other type of headache. The word tension describes the state of the muscle. It can be tensed, or contracted, as the result of a physical or emotional trigger.

The skull rests on the vertebra and, like other bones, the vertebra (spine) and neck are held in position by tendons, ligaments and many layers of muscle. These muscles and most other muscles in the body are part of the complex system of fully automatic reflexes that help to protect us against injury. For example, if you fracture your leg the muscles contract around the break and form a 'splint' to prevent movement and further injury. Often the pain from this splint is worse than the pain from the injury itself. Another example is the tightening of the abdominal muscles (this is called guarding) to protect internal organs when the appendix becomes inflamed.

In the same way, the contracted muscles which produce your headache, rather than a punishment, are an automatic protective measure which is really saying 'Don't abuse me'.

Emotional triggers

Emotional triggers which cause muscles in the head and neck to react are blushing when you are embarrassed and turning pale when you are afraid. You might ask why the muscles respond with pain when the trigger is emotional distress. The answer is that the muscles of the head and neck (and indeed other muscles) cannot differentiate between emotional and physical strain, so a bone out of alignment, a strained posture, fear, a bad marriage, overwork, depression or a large gas bill could all prompt the protective 'splinting' reaction. Perhaps if we were animals we would retreat into our shells or stick our heads in the sand. Instead of that we don the 'armour' of tension – a veritable iron helmet and shoulder protector.

Physical triggers

- *Injury*: explained above.
- *Posture*: holding the body in strained positions: standing badly,

12

sitting unsupported, unbalancing the head, for example.

- *Bedtime television watching*: the head propped forward while you peer at the screen.
- *Looking down while reading*: putting a strain on the neck.
- *Painting a ceiling*, or working in awkward situations such as under a car or the kitchen sink.
- *Facial mannerisms*: frowning, squinting, jaw-clenching.
- *Dental tension*: prolonged chewing (gum), abnormal chewing to avoid sensitive teeth, jaw problems, teeth-grinding.
- *Infections*: swelling.
- *Eye strain*: fatigue in the muscles surrounding the eye.
- *Spectacle problems*: pulling the head back to look through half-glasses or bifocals.

Neck problems and headaches

Muscle-contraction headaches can accompany arthritis of the neck (cervical spondylitis). Patients often say their pain is due to this condition in a resigned way that suggests they are doomed to headaches for the rest of their life. This is not necessarily the case. It puzzles me that this diagnosis is so often made without any physical examination or X-ray. Is it perhaps that in persons over 45 wear and tear in the neck joints is sometimes assumed when it is not actually present? It would seem difficult to differentiate in the absence of a history of arthritis and at least a physical examination, between cervical spondylitis and muscle spasm in the neck muscles from an emotional or physical trigger.

Arthritis

Arthritis is an inflammation of the joints. Any joint in the body can be affected. There are several types but the most common ones are osteoarthritis and rheumatoid arthritis. Osteoarthritis is by far the most common and the incidence increases with age – wear-and-tear arthritis. Rheumatoid arthritis can develop in young people and is by far the more serious condition. It can cause severe pain and deformity leading to disability.

When there is osteoarthritis in the neck there is an increased likelihood of developing muscle-contraction headaches. This could be another 'splinting' reaction and also a response to the pain. Portions of the damaged bone can press on nerves and pinch them. The nerves react with compression, irritation and eventually inflammation. This can also happen with a slipped disc. The shock absorber or cushion between the vertebrae presses on the nerve, causing pain. Both osteoarthritis and a slipped disc can cause neurological symptoms such as numbness, weakness and tingling. When the cervical spine is involved this will be felt in the arms. As has been said, a person who has a painful physical focus is also more likely to be affected by emotional triggers – fear of the pain, low mood, frustration. This adds to the tension in the neck and thus causes more headaches.

Combination headaches

The headaches of the chronic sufferer may have both muscular and vascular (blood-vessel) components. Superimposed on their tension headaches they can suffer periodic migraine headaches. It can also happen the other way around; migraine sufferers can get 'ordinary tension headaches'. This mechanism is easier to understand, since the migraine sufferer can induce tension in the neck muscles through fear of moving the head. Injuries to the neck such as whiplash and congenital cervical spine problems are also causes of tension headaches.

Headaches caused by movement and posture

The exertional headache

This headache may have a sharp or stabbing quality and may last minutes or hours. People who are prone to headaches often suffer from this type. Physical exercise, lifting, stooping or even coughing, sneezing or yawning (which can also be a sign of low blood sugar or air hunger) can bring it on. Perhaps the headache associated with lovemaking also comes into this category.

Orgasmic headache

These are thought to be caused by an increase in blood pressure, which causes the blood vessels in the head to dilate. The pain can be intense and may appear just before or during orgasm. It can last for minutes or several hours. The following may help:

14

- two aspirin or paracetamol tablets before intercourse;
- a cool shower or ice pack to the back of the neck before intercourse;
- keeping as cool as possible during lovemaking;
- keeping the head as elevated as possible during lovemaking;
- a strong cup of coffee before intercourse could constrict the blood flow to the head.

Hairdressing headache

Some people get a dull headache after a visit to the hairdresser's, where they have held their head back over the basin for a shampoo. The headache arrives later in the day or the following morning. It can be avoided by bending forward over the basin.

What happens when the muscles in the head or neck are tense?

A mechanical failure develops which produces brain symptoms and local symptoms. The blood vessels constrict, the brain chemistry is altered because it can't function properly without an adequate blood flow, and pain and stiffness develop in the muscles (the fibres contract) because they are not being adequately nourished either; another reason for the pain is a build-up of the waste products of metabolism in the tissues.

Stopping the washing-machine mid-cycle

A healthy lymphatic system takes nourishment to the cells and then carries the garbage away. When the muscles are contracted the waste products are trapped in the tissues and crystalline deposits form in the muscles in the same way that soap deposits would collect in your shirt if you repeatedly washed it and turned the dial to spin dry before it had been through the rinsing cycle. These deposits are another source of pain, although the sufferer, because of restricted movement, may not realize just how much trouble the garbage in the muscles is causing until a downward pressure is exerted on the muscles covering the shoulder-blades. This is often very painful and if the condition becomes chronic the tissues can become inflamed and swollen.

In muscular-contraction headaches the blood vessels are usually constricted, but like any other muscular tube under strain, periodic striving to correct the position can cause dilation which would be felt as sharp stabs of pain just as in intestinal colic.

Features of a tension headache

Distribution of pain

The pain is usually dull on the top of the head, extending from the forehead like a tight band and can go down the back of the head, behind the ear, into the jaw and across the face. The muscles at the base of the skull are often very tender on pressure. The pain can extend further, to the neck, shoulders and upper back.

When does the pain start?

It can come at any time of the day but rarely starts in the night. It usually affects both sides and can produce a feeling of a weight on the top of the head or a tight band around the head accompanied by a 'spacy' feeling. Sufferers can go to bed with a headache and wake up with the same headache. This is more common in people who are anxious and depressed. Their subconscious works away all night trying to help resolve their emotional conflicts and the result is that they awake as tense as when they retired to bed. It is more usual, however, for the pain to start in the morning and gradually worsen as the day progresses, with sleep bringing some measure of relief.

How long does the headache last?

It can last hours, days or even weeks if nothing is done about it. It is easy to understand why these headaches can be protracted. When the muscles are habitually overstimulated they become so contracted that merely switching off by reading, watching television or sleeping is not enough to allow them to rest in their lengthened state. The muscles need practical help in the form of stretching, massage, acupressure or other hands-on treatment, or the person might resort to painkillers, muscle relaxants or alcohol. The drawbacks of using drugs and alcohol are discussed later.

Who suffers from this type of headache?

Both sexes (in about equal proportions) and all ages. They usually start in early adult life although 10–20 per cent of sufferers have their first attacks in childhood (Saper and Magee, 1978).

Children and tension

One might imagine that children would escape tension in the head, neck and shoulders, because they were supple and active and don't have the responsibilities of adult life. This is definitely not so; life is different but just as difficult for them. The neuroses of later life are incubated during the early years. Children often find it difficult to express emotional pain and this can be missed by the adults around them. It is impossible to have all our needs met even if we are born into loving, stable families – the world is a fearful place. We react to this fear by tightening our muscles or 'armouring'. This practical mechanism allows us to hold in our fear, frustration, anger, grief, sadness or any other hurtful emotion. Thus the foundation stone of neurosis is laid. For more about this see Trickett (1989).

In children, physical triggers causing muscle tension include the persistent cough which keeps the shoulders raised, badly placed desks and pushing the head forward to peer at the blackboard. Sleeping on the stomach can put a strain on the neck, as can being carried on the mother's hip and having to turn the head in one direction to see the world. Sadly, also, children often spend long hours in front of badly positioned TV sets or lying on the floor lifting the head up to play computer games.

Appearance of a person with a tension headache

They are usually very pale, because of the constriction of the blood vessels, the face lacks expression and the eyes look dull. The sufferer often looks detached, as though they are not quite with you. If there are sinus problems in addition to the tension headache there can be dull red patches over the cheek-bones and fluid retention around the eyes. Sometimes the face can look puffy. This is probably because of congestion due to the tight muscles impeding the lymph drainage from the head. Furrowing of the brow can also be a feature.

Symptoms which can accompany the headache

- Visual disturbances: these are not as dramatic as in migraine sufferers, but they can occur in tension headaches, usually in the form of blurred vision or, if it is severe, there can be altered perception. In a *hallucination* the person sees something that is not there – for example a pink elephant. In *altered perception* the person sees what is there – for example, a flower on a curtain may appear like a face.

- Pain in the neck, shoulders and back.
- Bloating of the stomach or bowel and wind. Often the passing of wind is the first sign that the headache is abating. Nausea and loss of appetite are often part of the symptom picture, or craving for foods not normally a part of the sufferer's diet.
- Shakiness and lack of muscular coordination: for example, difficulty gripping a pen or clumsiness and regularly dropping things.
- Fatigue and lack of interest in things normally enjoyed.
- Wobbly legs: feelings of not quite knowing where the ground is or of walking on eggshells.
- Dizziness, especially when turning the head.
- Irritability, anxiety, depression and feeling of unreality; for example, walking into the kitchen and it being unfamiliar; or depersonalization – when a person looks into the mirror and they know intellectually it is their image they see but somehow they look different, rather like a distorted image in a mirror at a funfair.
- Difficulty in breathing through the nose – mild hyperventilation.

Some of these symptoms might seem rather remote from the site of pain, but because they happen with such monotonous regularity, most people are very accurate about their symptom picture; and the same symptoms crop up again and again in large numbers of people.

The pain is less disabling than migraine. Most sufferers continue working through these headaches and rarely retreat to bed during the day. Many people accept their headaches almost as a way of life.

Are your muscles tense?

1 Tilt your head back and gaze at the ceiling. If this makes you feel dizzy the muscles of your neck could be part of your problem.
2 (Not for those with back problems.) Standing up and keeping your knees straight, see how far you can easily reach to your toes. Do not strain. If you cannot reach much below your knees then your back muscles are tense.

Typical experiences

Woman of 30

I had been having tension headaches for almost a year before I pinpointed what they were. I could carry on working but the headaches were beginning to get me down. It was all a bit of a mystery to me. If I had been anxious or depressed perhaps it would have been easier to understand. My life was going well. I had a new job, which was exciting and hectic, I moved to a better flat and bought a car. For the first few months I was on cloud nine. Then began what I can only describe as a feeling of fullness and nausea in the muscles of my neck and shoulders. The headaches started with feelings of my head being heavy and sometimes I had an overwhelming desire to go to sleep. Over the weeks it changed to a dull continual ache in the whole of my head and the right side of my neck and my right shoulder. A couple of times I thought I was getting flu but nothing developed. I then thought it was perhaps sinus headaches and tried some nasal decongestant tablets from the chemist's. These didn't help much so I saw my doctor. He said they were tension headaches and gave me painkillers. If I took them regularly throughout the day they did ease the pain but I did not like the feeling that went with them. They gave me a muzzy head and I felt tired. I stopped taking them after a few weeks. The headaches came back with full force and I did not get any relief or real insight into how I was bringing them on until the computers were off at work for two days following a weekend. During this enforced break my head cleared considerably. I had to admit that my boyfriend was right when he argued that it was the stress at work. I could not see this because I was thoroughly enjoying my job. I made a big effort to slow down: got up earlier and made time to have breakfast and pack food for lunch (there was no canteen at this job and I had been having a doughnut or sausage roll for lunch). My boyfriend massages my neck and shoulders with olive oil each night and I made a neck pillow from a rolled towel bound with a crêpe bandage. I stretched my neck regularly throughout the day and tried not to hunch my shoulders. Making sure I did not sit for any more than 45 minutes at my desk at work without having a walk around the office was the hardest thing. I felt rather silly always wandering around. If I work late too often or get myself uptight about anything the pain comes back but generally it is very much better and I feel in control now – it does not control me. The muscles in my neck and shoulder are still very tender and this reminds me that the headaches are still lurking in the background and will come back if I am not vigilant.

This experience illustrates that the nervous system not only cannot distinguish between physical and emotional triggers for headaches but also that it does not matter whether the cause is painful or pleasurable. The new job and exciting life caused the problem.

Woman of 43

I had never been a headachy person so I was mystified by the severe headaches which appeared out of the blue. I felt sick and shaky with them and my neck and shoulders ached and felt like a ton weight. Paracetamol took the edge off it but the relief did not last long. They were worse at the end of the day and I began to dread going to work.

After about three months I went to an osteopath to see if there was something wrong with my neck. He said the muscles were in spasm and asked me if I had been doing anything different over the months. I could not think that I had. I was in the same job and had not had any added strain. I worked as a secretary but my desk was in good light by a window. When he asked me how long it was since I had been to have my eyes tested I said it could not be anything to do with my eyes because I had bought new glasses about four months earlier. He swooped on this and asked if they were half-glasses. They were, in fact. I had chosen them because the plastic frames had been making a red mark on my nose and I thought these would be lighter. He then explained what I had been doing – pulling my head back to see the full screen of my word processor through the lens. He pulled my head into that position and my muscles felt really sore. I could not imagine how I had missed this. He adjusted the bones of my neck and I went back for a few sessions of massage with an electrical thing and the headaches have gone. I went back to my old glasses until I got some fibreglass full-framed ones. My vanity over a red mark on my nose had caused months of headaches!

Man of 47

My job entails hours of driving and I had blamed the fumes of the traffic and irregular hours for my persistent headaches. I had been to the doctor to have my blood pressure checked. He said I was a bit overweight but everything else seemed fine and advised me to cut down on drinking and take more exercise. I was a regular drinker but not vast quantities. I did this and started walking more but there was no improvement. I had my eyes tested and they were unchanged since the last visit.

If it had not been for the back pain I would probably still be having the headaches. I turned to open the fridge and my back went. It was excruciating. The doctor seemed unconcerned. He told me to lie flat for a few days and gave me muscle relaxants. I had never had back pain before and was convinced that there was something very seriously wrong. Within a week I felt much better and went back to work. On my first long drive my head throbbed and I was aching all down my back. My neck felt barely able to support my head.

It was my wife's lack of sympathy that finally made me do something. She said living with me was miserable and although she did not actually voice it I felt she was hinting that she would leave me. She had left me briefly years before. She insisted I went to a stress management course.

The first evening was a waste of time but the second was on stress caused by driving. This did make sense. The instructor showed what happened when the head was pushed forward for long hours to peer at the road. I realized that I had been doing this and that my seat was not right. I bought a back support (I am not very tall) and put a cushion in the small of my back. I could feel the difference almost at once. I have also become more aware of how I move and how I sit when relaxing. I began to eat more fruit and vegetables and lost half a stone in weight. I still get the odd headache but they are nothing like what they were.

This account highlights the fact that keeping the head in an unbalanced position for protracted periods throws the whole spine out of alignment – the tension goes to the neck and shoulders, and then travels down the back.

Woman of 60

I had put up with headaches for years and if I had not developed panic attacks I might still be having them. The headaches I had coped with, but the panic attacks sent me rushing to the doctor. They were so terrifying, I did not think of them as panic attacks. I felt as though I was dying or at least had some very serious illness. The doctor tried to reassure me but I was not convinced. He said that they were just a sign that I had been under stress. That was what I could not understand because it was the first time for years that I was *not* under stress – my time was my own since my invalid mother had gone to live with my sister. I was really happy about her being there and was enjoying reading and gardening and, best of all, a full night's sleep. It was all very puzzling. I searched the bookshops for information on panic attacks and had to admit that the doctor must have been right – the feelings I was getting, palpitations, sweating, feeling unable to breathe and desperate feelings of fear and feeling that something dreadful was going to happen were all there. It said they were more common in people who had symptoms of tension such as headaches and neck aches. I had thought that perhaps the headaches were due to an old whiplash injury. I had never felt particularly tense and I certainly did not feel unhappy.

The headaches and panic attacks persisted and it was not until I was afraid to go out that the doctor arranged for a community psychiatric nurse to come to see me. It was her explanation which finally convinced me I was not dying of something terrible. She explained that after years of strenuous activity looking after Mother, suddenly my body had no need of the adrenalin which had kept me going and that my body was still producing so much that it flooded over the top causing panic attacks. She taught me how to calm down, breathe slowly and let my muscles relax. She also accompanied me on shopping trips until I could go out alone. I don't get headaches now and the panic attacks have decreased to just an odd flutter in the stomach now and then.

This experience is an example of how after years of pressing the panic button to produce lots of adrenalin, the body is not able to adjust overnight to you saying that it is time to relax – the panic is over.

Woman of 34

I had suffered headaches since I was about four years old. My mother did not take much notice of them – she just gave me junior aspirin and told me to lie down or go out in the fresh air. I had the feeling that she did not really believe me, and as I got older I felt she thought I was inventing them to avoid school or duck some chore I did not want to do. This was probably the case sometimes but I know I did not imagine the headaches because they also often prevented me doing things I wanted to do. I can still remember the weight at the back of my neck and the feeling that my arms would not move properly. The headaches also made my eyes hurt and sometimes I felt sick. Looking back I can see I was a loving child, very anxious to please, lonely and frightened. My parents rowed constantly and although I never saw any violence I always worried in case they would hurt each other. I used to lie in bed when they presumably thought I was asleep and pull the covers over my head to shut out the noise of their shouting.

They were not bad parents and I'm sure they loved me, and still do, in their way, but they seemed totally aware of the effect their relationship had on me.

I stayed at home until I was 20 in the mistaken belief that my presence would somehow help the situation and also perhaps because I was nervous about moving away.

The headaches became worse after I left school. I did not have a job and spent a lot of time in the house.

When I finally decided to go to college (encouraged by my aunt) I moved as far away as I could. It was the best thing I ever did. My parents separated. It seemed that far from helping the situation I had kept it going. They were staying together until I left home.

The headaches completely vanished a couple of months after I left home. It was a really odd feeling, as though there was a space where the weight should have been.

I met a boy in the first week at university doing the same course. We now live together. At first I was very anxious about visiting home in the holidays but I have got over that now and I'm fine unless I have to see my parents together.

This young woman's story outlines how constant nagging fear at any age can trigger headaches – a purely emotional cause in an otherwise healthy person. Whatever the cause the physiological end result is the same.

Man of 52

I started having headaches a couple of weeks after I was made redundant. I think I was in a state of shock. I had worked for the same firm for 14 years, got up at the same time, met the same people every day and then suddenly it was all gone, and added to that I had the worry of how I was going to carry on paying my mortgage and supporting my family.

The pain started with a dull ache at the base of my skull which I could move with a couple of aspirins but when they got fiercer the pills did not work. They went on and on and I eventually went to the doctor. He said he could give me headache tablets but he felt the real trouble was depression and that he would rather give me antidepressants. I was very much against drugs and refused, and also refused his offer to see a counsellor. I felt I had to work it out for myself.

A month later I was glad to go back and take the antidepressants. I got up with a headache and went to bed with a headache. Things were going from bad to worse. I was very irritable and my wife was showing signs of strain.

I felt horrible for the first week on the pills. My headache was just the same and added to it I had a queer, other-worldly feeling. I was tempted to stop them but my wife encouraged me to carry on. The doctor did say it would be a few weeks before I felt the benefit. After a couple of weeks I was getting more sleep – not waking at the crack of dawn with thoughts rushing around in my head – and from then on things improved.

I have been on them eight weeks now and can't say I'm back to normal (how can I be without a job?) but things don't seem so black and my head is a great deal better. I don't intend to carry on with the pills long-term. I just need a rest to pull up and get myself motivated again. I am thinking of applying for a grant to start a small business.

This experience shows how headaches can start after a shock and can be very much part of anxiety and depression. Many people live in a permanent state of low-grade depression without even realizing what is wrong. They accept continual headaches and fatigue as a way of life and struggle on through the greyness, often fiercely denying that they are depressed. It is as though they accept the physical pain and it protects them from really looking at what is wrong in their lives. It could be an unhappy marriage or a job where they are completely unfulfilled or a situation where they continually subjugate their needs to the needs of others and underneath feel resentful and angry. Often looking at these issues and bringing them into the open is far more scary than covering them up with headaches.

5

Migraine: Common, classical, cluster headaches

Ten per cent of the population of the UK suffer from migraine. The condition affects both sexes, all age groups, 'civilized' and primitive peoples. Even babies can suffer from migraine. The word is often used to describe any severe headache which no one knows how to cure. The inaccuracy of this should become apparent as you read on.

Migraine in literature

Many writers have described their migraine attacks in their stories. They include Shakespeare, Anthony Trollope, G. K. Chesterton and Rudyard Kipling. Perhaps the most notable is Lewis Carroll – even his images suggest the visual disturbances of a migraine attack and this text often refers to the severe pain. Tweedledum comments in *Through the Looking Glass*, ' "I'm very brave, generally," he went on in a low voice: "only today I happen to have a headache." ' Tweedledum's heavy headgear is also an indication of what the writer is feeling. ' "Do I look very pale?" said Tweedledum, coming up to have his helmet tied on. (He *called* it a helmet, though it certainly looked much more like a saucepan.)'

The migraine attack

This could be said to be a collection of symptoms usually involving severe recurring headache, thought to be vascular (constriction usually followed by dilation of the blood vessels to the brain) in origin, in a person where full investigations fail to reveal an organic cause and where typical symptoms accompany different phases of the attack. For example, mood changes in the prodromal (warning) phase, followed by severe headache, with or without digestive symptoms such as nausea, vomiting, bloating and diarrhoea, and also neurological symptoms (in classical migraine), which include visual disturbances, paraesthesia (pins and needles), clumsiness or transient paralysis. Recovery is usually after the 'hangover' phase, in which the sufferer feels exhausted. The sequential nature of each set of symptoms plus the length of time of each phase clearly distinguishes it from other types of headaches such as muscular (tension) headaches, although it is possible for a migraine sufferer also to be prone to tension headaches, and at times they might even coexist.

The term 'migraine' is of French origin, but its root is from the Greek term *hemicrania*, meaning affliction of half of the head.

What's in a word?

Not a lot in this case! How can one word describe several distinct conditions which constitute the phenomenon of migraine, some of which can bring a plethora of frightening, disabling and bizarre symptoms. Any new sufferers who have been diagnosed as having migraine and who seek confirmation and reassurance from a dictionary are likely to be disappointed, particularly if they have the type of migraine which involves neurological symptoms.

Attitudes to migraine

Migraine attacks have been recorded historically for over two thousand years. It is astonishing that for a condition which has been around for so long and affects 10 per cent of people in the United Kingdom alone, there is limited understanding and still no medical cure. Prescribed drugs help some people to lead near-normal lives but many of them bring their own problems. What is even more unfathomable than the limited help available is the archaic attitude towards the condition. It is generally regarded just as a tiresome headache, visited upon tiresome people, who through their tiresomely regular visits to the surgery, their frequent absences from work ('she's/he's having another one of her/his migraines'), their frequent retreats to lie down in a darkened room, deliberately make life tiresome for those around them. If your pancreas fails to secrete insulin and you develop diabetes you are unlikely to encounter any problems – swift diagnosis, effective treatment, continued support. The same happens if you develop another 'respectable' condition like pernicious anaemia – injections of vitamin B12, continued care – no hint that you are malingering. Better still if some part of you can be replaced, removed or treated with some high-tech medicine – all very respectable.

Why is migraine such a poor relation in medicine?

Firstly because it is non-life-threatening, and secondly because it involves changes in brain chemistry and therefore alteration in mood and behaviour. When a spanner is thrown into the works of the great neurochemical factory, the brain (about which science admits it still has a lot to learn), there is bound to be a multiplicity of symptoms. Perhaps it is these which lead non-sufferers to believe that migraine is a rather nasty headache – but everyone gets a headache at some time! – with a hint of hypochrondria.

What happens during an attack

Migraine could be described as a disorder of arousal. Placid people are less likely to suffer but are not immune. The brain stem, the oldest part of the brain, controls the autonomic nervous system, which oversees body functions such as the muscular activity of the digestive system, breathing, circulation and sensory perceptions, sound, touch, taste, hearing and smell. It also includes the reticular activating system (RAS). This mechanism determines how much stimulation is allowed to reach the brain. For example, two people who go to the same party will have RAS systems which react differently. A has an RAS system which is partly closed but still alert enough to react if there was danger such as a fire in the building. B has an RAS system which is wide open and reacts much more to the stimuli around him. A is likely to go home and relax into a sound sleep. B is likely to be overstimulated long after leaving the noise and excitement of the party. The inability to relax might make him resort to tranquillizers or alcohol to induce sleep. A and B have both had the same stimulation but react differently.

The lymbic system is controlled by the hypothalamus, which prompts the release of chemicals from the pituitary and adrenal glands. It is unable to distinguish between the signals of fear or pain and pleasure or excitement. When the senses are not being stimulated the hypothalamus reduces the supply of stress hormones and secretes endorphins which produce a state of relaxation. The hypothalamus has a high concentration of the neurotransmitter serotonin (see p. 37), which is a chemical messenger between nerve cells.

Taking your migraine to the doctor

Doctors' reactions to migraine vary a great deal. A consultation can be caring and very thorough, or it can be caring but lacking in helpful information or treatment, or sadly, as is so often the case, it can be dismissive and hurtful. This may be because the doctor is irritated with the patient for making a fuss about what he sees as 'just a headache', or it can be that the practitioner is angry with himself over his own inadequacy in the management of migraine – he has nothing other than a prescription for painkillers, which he knows are of limited use, to offer the patient.

Typical experiences of a consultation

I was very frightened when I arrived at the surgery utterly convinced I was going to die from a brain tumour. I felt something serious must be going wrong in my head to cause such excruciating pain and to affect my vision and speech. After a detailed histoy, including questions about my relatives, the doctor said he was almost certain that my problem was migraine, but this could not be confirmed until I had been examined and had undergone some routine tests. *Migraine!* I listened to this with a mixture of disbelief and relief. The doctor said he was referring me to a neurologist at the Migraine Clinic, who he felt sure would confirm the diagnosis.

I left the surgery feeling better although not totally convinced. I was given a prescription for painkillers and a leaflet about migraine. The leaflet aroused my fears again. It did not describe anything like I was experiencing. It was brief and mentioned more about triggers than symptoms. I felt desperate to see the symptoms I was having under the heading 'Migraine'. I think that would have convinced me.

The doctor was very kind and reassuring but I still wondered if he was holding something back from me. In retrospect I realize I was in such a state of anxiety it would have taken a lot to put my mind at ease.

I have had migraine for seven years. The need to take more and more time off work drove me to see my GP. It was a waste of time. I felt anxious and rushed as I tried to explain the symptoms, worried that I was leaving something vital out. He looked at my notes all the time and I wondered if he was listening to me.

After taking my blood pressure and looking into my eyes he said, you have had headaches a long time. There is nothing to suggest they are anything more than migraine. Would you like some painkillers? I was in and out in five minutes.

After years of unhelpful, dismissive consultations with my doctor I gave up making appointments. I always felt worse when I came out, almost as if I were to blame for the pain. It was when I had an attack at work and saw the works' doctor that I got some help. He gave me an injection to stop the vomiting and made me lie down. He asked me to make an appointment to see him the following week for a chat. I had more information in that 20-minute conversation than I had ever had. No one had ever explained what happens during an attack and what changes I could make in my life-style to lessen attacks. He recommended some reading and gave me an address to send off for a relaxation tape. I walked out on air – I had previously thought of migraine as something one just 'had' – something that you just had to live with.

Types of migraine

The condition described as *common* migraine accounts for 80 per cent of migraine attacks. The rarer *classical* migraine has been recorded historically for over 2,000 years and has a more compli-cated, well-defined symptom picture. Both types usually share the symptom of a severe headache. *Cluster* headache is rarer and can be easily distinguished from the other types.

The stages of a migraine attack
1 Warning or pre-headache phase.
2 The aura (classical migraine).
3 The headache.
4 The postdromal or 'hangover' phase.

Common migraine

The warning phase

The pre-headache phase is seen in both common and classical migraine although it is not experienced by all common migraine sufferers. It may last for a few hours or even for several days before an attack. The phase may include:

- mood changes
- tension
- irritability
- confusion
- mental dullness
- vertigo
- fainting
- fatigue

- weight gain
- nausea
- hunger
- stuffy nose
- raised blood pressure
- extra energy
- euphoria

The headache phase

The pain can last for a few hours to three days and is described by most sufferers as hot and pulsating; it affects the head, face, jaw and sometimes the neck and shoulder area. The latter may be the result of holding the head in a fixed position, since the slightest movement or coughing or sneezing can increase the pain. The pain may be worse on one side and attacks frequently occur around the time of menstruation. The sufferer usually notices the headache on waking, although it can actualy wake them up.

Vomiting, diarrhoea and constipation are frequently present, and these can lead to dehydration. The sufferer often describes their affliction as 'sick headaches'. Sufferers may feel hot/cold/sweaty, but a recent study showed that recorded temperatures were normal (Blau, 1991). Acute sensitivity to light, sound and smell can also be present. Neurological symptoms are rare in common migraine.

Abating of headache

Symptoms improve with time and loss of body fluids through vomiting, diarrhoea, increased flow of urine, tears, sweating or streaming nose.

The hangover phase

The sufferer often feels drained of energy and has to move slowly. Even thinking can be an effort.

Classical migraine

The pre-headache phase

Typically, classical migraine sufferers report that the aura is the first sign of an attack, but in some people the pre-headache phase is also experienced. This is sometimes called the 'prodrome', from the Greek *prodromos* meaning 'coming before'. The experience can be one of fearfulness and depression, or of feeling very well, full of energy and creativity.

The aura

This is thought to arise from disturbances in the blood flow to the head. The symptoms depend on which part of the brain is affected. They can be frightening and bizarre and people often think they are going mad or having a stroke. The aura may only last for 15 to 20 minutes before the onset of the headache.

Visual disturbances

hypersensitivity to light } these appear in both types of
blurred vision   } migraine, but are not the aura
double vision   } symptoms; they are noted here for
                                        } convenience

partial blindness
blind spot in one or both eyes (scotoma)
tunnel vision
figures appear elongated or shortened
spots or sparkling shapes or glare

Visual disturbances often cause clumsiness and bumping into things. There can also be a distortion of body image or the sufferer may feel that part of the body is 'not there'.

The headache phase

Sensory disturbances

- acute sensitivity to slightest noise
- ringing in ears

- altered taste sensation
- acute sensitivity to touch.

Neurological symptoms

- lack of coordination
- weakness in limbs
- tingling
- transient paralysis
- inability to grip
- inability to find words
- speech problems.

Organic and circulatory symptoms

- nausea
- abdominal pain
- gut rumbling
- belching
- increased urination
- thirst
- diarrhoea
- pseudo-angina
- cold hands and feet
- vertigo
- fainting.

Psychological symptoms

- tension
- feelings of dread
- confusion
- memory loss.

Visible signs

- pallor
- flushing
- bloodshot eyes
- yawning
- sweating.

The headache phase can last from four to 72 hours in adults and less in children. The pain may initially be unilateral but as it worsens it can spread to a deep throbbing pain all over the head, behind the eyes, in the ear and jaw, and the neck and shoulders. Generalized aches and pains can also be present, plus nausea, vomiting and prostration.

The post-headache phase

The person can be exhausted, confused and depressed, or sluggish, with stiff, sore muscles. Large amounts of urine can be passed and sometimes there is abnormal appetite or food cravings. Severe diarrhoea can also be a feature. A minority of people feel 'cleansed' and in high spirits. This may be due partly to relief that the attack is over, or there may be a biochemical reason similar to the sudden 'lift' some women feel after a period.

After a severe migraine attack

As Mary K. Henneberger points out, in a reprint from the *Newsletter* of the National Headache Foundation, Chicago, USA, the aftermath of a severe migraine is generally overlooked in headache literature and frequently ignored in treatment. Aching limbs, neck, shoulders and back may persist for several days and a deep pain or sore spot in the back, described by Oliver Sachs as the post-migraine 'bruise' (Sachs, 1970), may be a source of discomfort for several days. Rest, the application of heat and analgesics may bring comfort.

Some simple measures to try

The 'pale' phase

Initially, when the blood vessels are constricted, the following may help:

- Lie flat to increase circulation to head; raise feet on pillows.
- Apply covered hot-water bottle to back of neck or hot lavender compress to forehead (five drops of essential oil of lavender – or any oil recommended by aromatherapist or book – in a bowl of hot water). Have two washcloths and change the cloth as soon as it cools.
- Massage scalp around the base of the skull and the neck, and gently move the shoulders.

- If well enough to stand, have a warm shower and hold the shower head close to the back of the neck.

The 'hot' phase

When the blood vessels dilate the tissues become engorged with blood and swell. Try:

- Lying or sitting propped up with the head well supported to decrease circulation to head.
- Apply ice pack to nape of neck and washcloths which have been in cold water (add ice from freezer), to forehead.
- Keep the rest of the body cool.
- Get someone to massage your feet or rest them on a covered hot-water bottle.
- Apply Tiger Balm (available from health stores or Asian stores) or Oil of Olbas (widely available in pharmacists) to neck and forehead. Both of these have a cooling effect.
- Have an ionizer as near your face as possible (see p. 111).
- If you can get off the bed, have a cool shower or Epsom salts bath. This will help to remove excess water from the body. Large packs of Epsom salts are available from pharmacies. Use three cupfuls in warm water. Apply cool washcloth to head.

Drugs used for migraine

This is a matter for you to discuss with your doctor and there is no doubt that for some people acute medication at times is the only effective treatment. There are, however, often unwanted side-effects and it is better to find out what is triggering your migraines rather than just treat the symptoms. Any drug taken for headaches suppresses the body's natural pain-relieving substances and if you are cutting down or cutting out medication, for a time your headaches will increase in intensity (Walker, 1993). This is the analgesic rebound effect. To cut down slowly and help the body to detoxify is the only way. There is no short cut.

Before discussing some of the drugs which can induce headaches, I must stress once again that any medication you are on for any condition should not be cut down or stopped without consulting your medical practitioner.

Drugs which cause headaches and migraine

A headache is one of the first signs to indicate you have taken a substance which the body regards as a poison. To list all the drugs where headaches are a side-effect would be to reproduce half of the *British National Formulary*. Special mention could be made of one of the antidepressant drugs, fluoxetine (Prozac) which, although it has been used to relieve migraine in some subjects, has also been found to produce it in a person who has never experienced a migraine attack before (Larson, 1993).

Common drugs which can cause headaches

Some common drugs dilate the blood vessels which supply the brain and therefore produce symptoms like the engorgement phase of migraine. When they are withdrawn a rebound constriction of the blood vessels can also be a cause of headaches.

- caffeine
- alcohol
- evening primrose oil
- vitamin B3
- tranquillizers and sleeping pills (benzodiazepines)
- monoamine oxidase inhibitor antidepressants
- nicotine.

Drugs used for migraine which may produce headaches in non-sufferers

- tricyclate antidepressants
- the contraceptive pill
- hormone replacement therapy
- non-steroidal anti-inflammatory drugs
- ergotamine.

Food triggers

Amines

These are substances necessary for brain and blood-vessel function. Some are found in food, others are manufactured in the body. They serve as neurotransmitters and a disturbance in the normal balance can cause disorders such as depression, Parkinson's disease and migraine.

Serotonin

This is an important nitrogen-containing amine and is found in a variety of tissues, including the brain. Since it constricts some blood vessels and contracts others it is not surprising that it is thought to play a key role in the production of headaches and migraine. Like other brain amines such as noradrenalin, it not only determines the size of blood vessels, but also controls mood and sleep patterns. Low levels of serotonin have been found in people who have committed suicide. High levels are known to cause mania, headaches and other problems.

The level of serotonin drops dramatically at the onset of a migraine attack, the constricted blood-vessel stage, and presumably rises rapidly with the dilation phase. Vomiting lowers serotonin levels. This could be why some people (particularly children) induce vomiting to relieve their headache. When the balance of amines is altered in the body a migraine can be triggered. When looking for the food that is triggering your migraine, remember it could be that it is the total amount of amines you are including in your diet rather than one specific food such as cheese or chocolate. Sensitivity to amine-rich foods is generally recognized by the medical profession as a trigger in migraine, although food intolerances (the leaky-gut syndrome, p. 57) as a cause of health problems is still a contentious issue in general practice.

Amine-rich foods

Dairy products

Cheese – particularly mature cheeses such as Stilton, Brie and Camembert – yogurt and sour cream. There seems to be divided opinion about milk; cottage and cream cheese are generally thought not to be a problem.

Meat

- pork
- game
- smoked meats
- offal.

Fish

- pickled and preserved fish.

Yeast extracts

- Marmite
- Vegemite
- miso
- soy sauce

37

- some stock cubes
- some packet soups
- some gravy powders.

Fruit and vegetables

- spinach
- citrus fruits (particularly oranges)
- bananas
- figs
- plums
- pineapples
- raisins
- avocados
- sauerkraut
- broad beans
- soya beans
- onions.

Products containing vinegar

- pickles
- relishes
- salad dressings
- sauces.

Chocolate

- confectionery
- chocolate desserts
- chocolate drinks.

Alcohol

All alcoholic drinks, particularly red wines, beer, sherry and some white wines. The effects of alcohol can be twofold: dilating the blood vessels and raising the amine levels. You can also be allergic to the corn in whisky, the hops in beer and the grapes or congeners in wine.

Monosodium glutamate headaches

A few years ago the 'Chinese restaurant syndrome' was described. It included headaches, often of the migraine type, sweating, hairs 'standing up on the back of the neck', burning in the chest, face, jaw, body and trunk. Symptoms usually occur within 15 to 20 minutes of eating. The trigger, monosodium glutamate, a flavour enhancer, is found in many products including dry-roasted peanuts, instant soups, instant gravies, some meat tenderizers and seasonings and some processed meats. Read labels carefully if you think you have had problems with this substance.

Nitrate headache

Nitrates produce dilation of blood vessels and in some people can produce a pounding headache. They have been used for centuries as a meat preservative. Some patients who take nitrate-containing drugs for angina complain of headaches. Foods containing nitrates include:

- tinned ham
- hot dogs
- corned beef
- salami

- bacon
- pepperoni
- smoked fish
- sausages.

Sleep patterns and migraine

Lack of sleep can trigger migraine and oversleeping at weekends can also produce a migraine. This could be due to low blood sugar, the post-stress migraine response or caffeine withdrawal (Couturier, 1993).

Post-stress migraine

This is very common and usually happens at weekends. A 14-year-old boy who had a migraine attack every weekend starting on Friday evenings and lasting until midday Sunday became completely migraine-free when he was moved from a rigid grammar school to the local comprehensive school. Many businessmen have weekend migraines.

Cluster headaches

This is a rarer type of headache which is easily distinguishable from other types of headache. They are often called histamine headaches because it is histamine which causes the pain and inflammation associated with allergic headaches. Men are more prone to this than women and it is usually middle-aged men who are affected, although it can start as early as the mid-twenties. Alcohol drinkers and smokers are much more at risk or even non-smokers who have to sit in a smoke-filled room. The name comes from the fact that the headaches appear in 'clusters' and the victim is perfectly well between attacks, which last for six to eight weeks. Alcohol is well known to precipitate an attack in a known sufferer.

It is characterized by severe unilateral pain in the eye and temple, often occurring in the night, and can be so intense that the sufferer bangs his head on a wall. The face is flushed and hot and the eye on the affected side is swollen and bloodshot; the pupil is small and there is often profuse tearing. The affected nostril either steams with clear fluid or is swollen and blocked. Fortunately the pain is of quite short duration, easing within the hour and leaving a dull ache around the eye which can last for several hours. This can happen several times a day. Without treatment the pain can return daily for several weeks.

Questions to ask yourself

- Did your headaches begin after the age of 25?
- Do your attacks occur at the rate of between one and six per day and continue for one to three months?
- Do you have eye and nose symptoms during the headache?
- Are you a smoker or drinker?
- Are you well between attacks?

Treatment

Inhalation of oxygen can abort an attack of this type of headache and GPs are able to prescribe this on the NHS. A large cylinder is needed because the flow-rate must be seven litres per minute (Blau, 1991).

Ergotamine tartrate can be used to prevent attacks although it is not without its risks and should not be prescribed for people with high blood pressure.

If you believe you have cluster headaches, it is essential to see your doctor to have the diagnosis confirmed; in addition, self-help methods to improve your general health can only be of value.

Migraine – the holistic approach

- Find the trigger.
- Boost your immune system and general health.
- Review your lifestyle and watch your stress levels.
- Look at your diet, alcohol intake, smoking habits, use of prescribed and over-the-counter drugs, and street drugs.
- Consider what you are opting out of when you have these migraines.
- Are you hanging on to negativity from the past?
- Are you full of pride and righteous indignation?
- Are your emotional needs being met?

- Are you afraid of death, of being alone?
- Do you ignore your spiritual needs?
- What about your feelings of self-worth?
- Investigate non-drug treatments.

Before you say 'but migraine is purely physical' – remember that **nothing is purely physical.**

6

Headaches caused by sinus problems

Television commercials would have us believe that all headaches with facial pain are due to sinus infections, and urge us to take their brand of antihistamine or decongestant. This is not so; there are numerous causes of facial pain with headaches. They include dental problems, temporo-mandibular joint (TMJ) problems and neuritis (nerve pains).

The sinuses are spaces in the bones of the skull which are filled with air from a small opening in the nose. The mucous membrane lining the nose is continuous with the lining of the sinuses and other structures connected with the nose, so infections in the nose can lead to infections of the eye, ear and (through the Eustachian tube) inner ear, and the mastoid process of the temporal bone, throat, bronchi and, although very rarely, the meninges (the outer covering of the brain) by way of the olfactory nerve.

There are various causes of sinus problems; these may be categorized as allergic, acute infective or chronic.

Allergic sinus headache

This is due to an allergic response inflaming the air inlet in the nose to the sinuses. It can be caused by inhalation of a substance (see p. 58) which causes swelling in the delicate nasal mucosa, or by eating or drinking something which has the same effect. The resulting headache is known as a vacuum headache. It is unlike hay fever in that it only rarely involves streaming eyes and nose. It does not seem to be the effect of local irritation, with rapid onset of sneezing and so on. It is, however, possible that the action of chewing food may transmit allergens into the nasal cavity, thus provoking a response in the nose directly (Brostoff and Gamlin, 1989).

Characteristics
- swelling inside the nose
- difficulty with breathing through the nose
- generalized headache, muzziness

- dizziness
- sudden mood change – anxiety, depression
- pain over the cheek-bones and eyebrows, and at the base of the nose.

The headache can be accompanied by:

- rapid pulse
- feeling weak and shaky
- swelling around the eyes
- hyperventilation
- bloated abdomen and wind
- fluid retention.

It is possible that the lining of the gut swells in the same way as the lining of the nose. This could account for the feeling of 'everything stopping' in the abdomen. Constipation and bloating and difficulty in passing even a soft stool are common, although in some cases diarrhoea can be present. Often the first sign that symptoms are abating can be the passing of wind and movement in the gut.

Feelings of anxiety or panic, with pins and needles or heavy limbs are often reported when the nose is blocked. Rapid shallow mouth-breathing during the night brings on the symptoms of hyperventilation (see pp. 99–100).

The symptoms may develop minutes after exposure or may take six or more hours to appear. Some symptoms such as restlessness and bloating may appear before the headache.

Appearance
Pale, puffy-faced and tired.

What to do to relieve symptoms

- If food intolerance has caused the reaction take a teaspoonful of bicarbonate of soda or, better still if you can get it, one teaspoonful each of bicarbonate of soda and potassium bicarbonate. (This is available from some chemists or you could try a health food store or nutritional supplier. 'Allergy Switch Off' is available from the Sanford Clinic – see Useful addresses.) Drink plenty of water; as soon as you can, eat a bland meal, for example rice, pasta or something you know you can tolerate. For some reason this seems to 'turn off' reactions in some people.

- To reduce swelling in nose – steam inhalations, steamy bath or shower followed by cool shower. (Allergies are always worse when you are hot.)
- Some people find taking an antihistamine helps.
- Sodium cromoglycate nasal spray (available over the counter as Resiston) helps some people, although it seems more effective in preventing a reaction (see p. 59).
- Take a homoeopathic remedy or paracetamol for the headache.
- Rest, with or without an ice pack (a packet of frozen peas wrapped in a thin cloth will do) on the head, forehead or over the bridge of the nose. Boots sell an ice pack with a cover.

In the longer term

- Have food and chemical allergy testing. Your doctor might be able to help you. If not, see an alternative practitioner who is knowledgeable on this subject. If you cannot afford this, read about elimination/rotation diets and pay attention to your general health. Read a candida questionnaire (see Trickett, 1994).
- Watch out for stress – you are far more likely to have reactions when your body is already overtaxed.

Case histories

Woman of 27

I was unwell for several weekends while staying with a friend before I associated it with travelling by train. My income had gone up so I began to travel by train instead of the coach. At first I thought I was allergic to her cats but knew they had never bothered me before. The only difference I could pinpoint was travelling by train. I don't know whether it's the air-conditioning or something from the brake fluid (I loathe the smell), but it was definitely something on the train because I have not had it again since I went back to coach travel.

When I look back I remember feeling restless on the train and my nose felt uncomfortably dry. By the time I arrived at my friend's my eyes were puffy and I felt muzzy-headed and tired. A couple of times she asked me if I had been having late nights. During the evening my head would ache, I would feel bloated and as though I was retaining fluid before a period. I would also feel very thirsty. The next day my sinuses would feel sore and I often felt dizzy and weak. It cleared up after I had been home for a couple of days.

Man of 42

This man had a long history of what he called sinus problems. After years of ineffective treatment with antihistamines, decongestants and occasionally antibiotics he realized that his problem was not due to infections or an allergic reaction to an outside allergen but to some reaction in his body chemicals. The attacks were always after he had been overworking or after a stressful event. He asked his doctor if it were possible to get inflammation in his body as a result of stress. He got no reply to this and was given a prescription for a nasal spray. There was never any nasal discharge or post-nasal drip – just a blocked nose, which he felt was swollen inside.

It would start with a feeling of being uptight and vaguely depressed and I would have difficulty thinking. Then my nose would feel blocked, my head muzzy, with pains across my cheekbones, and my stomach would feel bloated and uncomfortable. I would go off my food and feel unsteady on my legs. My neck and shoulders always felt very tense and my face would go pale and puffy. My wife said she always knew when it was coming on because I had dull red marks below my cheek-bones. I often felt as if I was going down with flu but there was never any sign of a temperature, although my face and head felt uncomfortably hot. The depression usually got worse and did not lift until the attack passed, which usually took three weeks no matter what I did. My sleeping was disturbed and I often woke up feeling slightly panicky, with pins and needles or a numb feeling in my arms.

The attacks became more frequent and my work and normally happy home life was being disrupted, so I had to slow down. I stopped working in the evenings, took a decent break at lunchtime and generally started to look after myself. Cutting down my

45

workload caused me some anxiety at first and I had to be disciplined about delegating or leaving things to the following day. I also put the answering machine on in the evenings. Nagging from my wife helped. She was getting very fed up with me being below par. After about six weeks I felt the effect and realized I was achieving more although I was working fewer hours. I have only had one 'sinus' attack in the past year and that was after a hectic business trip to Canada.

Infective sinus problems

Acute sinusitis is an infection of the lining of the nose and sinuses caused by bacteria, viruses or fungus (although this is not often looked for as a cause of sinus problems); it can spread to the throat and ears. It often appears about a week to ten days after a cold or flu as a secondary infection.

You can feel tired, lack concentration or have a feeling that your head is too heavy to be supported by your neck. Feeling vaguely anxious or depressed for no apparent reason, for a day or two before the attack really gets going, is common.

Symptoms
- fever
- severe headache, facial pain, pain at the base of the nose, pain at the back of the neck and sometimes into the shoulders
- dizziness
- severe facial pain when you bend your head forward – this can also make you feel nauseated
- blocked nose
- dry throat, coated tongue
- uneasy feeling in digestive tract
- inability to think clearly.

Appearance
The face can look normal or swollen and can either be pale with red patches over the cheeks or be generally flushed. The nose can be swollen, with redness over the bridge. There is often considerable puffiness around the eyes (which can be bloodshot) and the neck can also look puffy. Some sufferers are sensitive to noise and light and most people with this infection feel generally very miserable.

Treatment

The aims of treatment are:

- to prevent the infection spreading to throat, ears and chest;
- to reduce the temperature and ease discomfort;
- to reduce the swelling in the nose so as to aid the discharge of mucus and allow air to flow into the sinuses.

If your symptoms do not respond to rest, aspirin or paracetamol, plenty of hot drinks and steam inhalations, see your doctor or homoeopath, particularly if your throat or ears are also involved. The doctor may prescribe an antibiotic.

Avoiding the unwanted effects of antibiotics

Antibiotics do not discriminate: when they kill bacteria they also kill off the useful bacteria which control the ecology of the gut and the result can be that fungi such as *Candida albicans* proliferate and cause symptoms such as bowel disturbances, a sore mouth, thrush and itching around the anus and genitals. These problems can be prevented or minimized by using antifungal preparations and avoiding foods such as sugar and yeast which encourage fungal growth (see Trickett, 1994).

Steam inhalations

These reduce swelling in the nasal passages and allow the draining of mucus from the sinuses. Use one pint of near-boiling water with or without:

- one teaspoonful benzoin tincture (Friar's Balsam)
- a couple of menthol crystals
- five drops of Oil of Olbas (can be inhaled directly from the bottle or on a tissue).

Bend the head, covered with a towel, over the bowl and breathe in slowly through the nose until the steam has gone.

All the above are available from the pharmacist. Do not use them for babies or children.

Essential oils

Several oils, including pine, eucalyptus, lavender, ginger, pepper-mint and niaouli are helpful for sinusitis. It is important to note, however, that essential oils are potent medicines and should be used with care during pregnancy and for children. Seek the help of an aromatherapist or follow the instructions in a book on aromatherapy.

Ice packs

An ice pack to the head or nape of the neck can be soothing. Use for 20 minutes in any one hour. (But see Note below.)

Lavender compress

Use five drops of lavender oil in a bowl of warm water. Soak two thin cloths (small pieces of old cotton) in the bowl. Wring out one and allow to dry on the forehead; then replace with the second cloth.

Note While the application of an ice pack can relieve some headaches, a cold substance in the mouth can actually cause a so-called 'ice-cream headache'. This headache is fortunately brief, though intense. When a cold substance touches the roof of the mouth many of the cranial nerves are affected and a dull throbbing pain can radiate all around the head. Children often cry out in pain at the first large spoonful of ice-cream. It can be avoided if the mouth is cooled slowly by eating small, well-spaced quantities. A biting wind can also produce a headache, usually in the forehead, temples or base of the skull.

Acute sinusitis – quick reference

- Seek professional help if the symptoms do not respond to rest, paracetamol and fluids.
- Keep in a warm atmosphere. Make the room steamy with wet towels on the radiator or an electric kettle. Germs in the nose breed more rapidly in cold conditions. The moist atmosphere will make it easier to breathe.
- If you have to go out in cold weather wear a hat and cover your nose and mouth with a scarf.
- Rest as much as possible.
- Use small tissues for blowing the nose and discard immediately. Wash hands.
- Take up to 3 g of vitamin C daily if your digestion can cope with it. If not, eat fresh fruit and vegetables.
- You will need your energy to fight the infection, so don't overload your digestion. Eat small, easily digested meals.

- Restock the gut with good bacteria. Supplements containing acidophilus are available in health food stores but to be sure of a quality product it is better to order through a nutritional supplier. BioCare Ltd (see Useful addresses) supply Replete, a special intensive seven-day programme to follow antibiotic usage.

Case histories

Man of 43

Two weeks after an attack of flu I had acute sinusitis for the first time. It felt as bad as flu; I was utterly miserable. My face and head ached and I had a high temperature. I was given antibiotics and after about a week my nose streamed with a thick yellow discharge. This greatly relieved the pains in my head and face although I still felt weak and depressed. Part of the trouble was difficulty sleeping.

This is a typical experience of acute sinusitis as a secondary infection after flu or a cold.

Woman of 33

Two years after I had stopped taking diazepam (Valium) I was very pleased with myself but was feeling run-down. (I had been on Valium for ten years and was originally prescribed it for exam nerves.) I was getting repeated sinus and ear infections which were really making me feel low and I was having a lot of sick leave. I had severe facial pain and could not look down at the keyboard, my concentration was nil and I felt dizzy and unreal. My ear discharged a lot and it dried around my ear and on my face like a salt deposit. It made the skin sore. It persisted in spite of several antibiotics. Eventually the doctor sent off a swab to the hospital. When the result came back he said he was surprised to find it was a fungal infection. I did not know at the time but learned later (from a health magazine) that long-term tranquillizer use can put a strain on the immune system and fungal infections after withdrawal are common. I was given anti-fungal drops and tablets and felt much better after a few days, although it did come back when the treatment stopped. I had to have two further courses of treatment.

Chronic sinusitis

This is a debilitating condition which makes the sufferer feel miserable. The nose and sinuses are in a permanent state of inflammation and infection. This can give rise to the following symptoms:

- headaches and facial pain
- nose blocked or running with thick mucus
- post-nasal drip – mucus discharging behind the nose
- swollen nose and face
- snuffling
- loss of sense of smell
- enlarged lymph glands in neck
- recurrent ear, throat or chest infections
- digestive problems caused by swallowing mucus
- loss of appetite
- general fatigue with aching muscles due to toxins
- disturbed sleep
- cough due to post-nasal drip.

Treatment

The aims of treatment are:
- to build up the immune system to enable it to cope with infection;
- to reduce swelling in nose so as to allow mucus to drain;
- to prevent reinfection.

If this has been a long-term problem with you, ask your doctor for referral to an ear, nose and throat unit for investigation to rule out nasal polyps or any other condition. Nasal polyps are small grape-like swellings of the membrane formed by prolonged irritation.

- Avoid long-term use of nasal sprays, antibiotics, decongestants or antihistamines (see p. 59).
- Review your lifestyle – if you are stressed your immune system cannot recover.
- Review your diet – are you eating mucus-forming foods such as dairy produce and refined carbohydrate?
- Avoid smoky atmospheres.

- Have regular steam inhalations.
- Investigate the possible allergy/candida connection.
- Gargle with tea tree oil or Citricidal. (Tea tree oil is available from Thursday Plantation and Citricidal from Penny Davenport at New Nutrition. See Useful addresses.)
- Learn about nasal hygiene (p. 48).
- Change your toothbrush frequently.
- Get as much fresh air as possible.
- Buy an ionizer (p. 111) for your bedroom.
- If you don't improve with self-help methods, seek help from complementary medicine.
- Try sleeping with more pillows.

Case histories

Woman of 57

I had recurrent ear infections after my fourth child was born and have had chronic sinus problems since. I have had X-rays and years of treatment from the doctor but it never seemed to clear completely. My sister suggested garlic capules and cod liver oil. It worked wonders. I still have a bit of trouble in the winter but it is better than it has been for years. Some of my aches and pains have gone too.

Man of 45

Chronic catarrh had plagued me for years. Antibiotics and the nasal spray had stopped working. My digestion became a big problem and the hospital said it was irritable bowel syndrome. At the time I did not realize how this and the treatment I had been having for years for the sinus problem tied in together. The pills I was given for my gut did not seem to do anything and the high-fibre diet definitely made me worse. The whole of my abdomen was distended and I felt inflamed inside.

My wife had sent off to a candida helpline for information on thrush; she had had it off and on for years. There was a leaflet enclosed on irritable bowel syndrome. It was the first thing that had made sense. I changed my diet and sent away for the candida control packs (from Health Plus – see Useful addresses). I felt a bit rough at first but it was worth it. Part of it, I think, was that it seemed to unblock my nose and swallowing the mucus down the back made me feel sick. When this drained I felt much better. I am on my third month of treatment and feel a different person.

This is a very common experience. Treating fungal overgrowth in the bowel often clears long-term ear, nose, throat and chest problems. It can also help chronic skin problems including psoriasis. While many doctors who practise nutritional medicine believe there is a direct link to fungal infections and psoriasis, conventional medicine favours the view that since the skin and gut come from the same part of the foetus, food intolerance is a more likely cause. It is estimated that 25 per cent of eczema sufferers and 20–25 per cent of psoriasis sufferers are milk intolerant (*British Medical Journal*, 1968). Many people on candida diets exclude all diary products.

Grapefruit-seed extract – a natural antibiotic

Grapefruit-seed extract (Citricidal) is an inexpensive, safe addition to your medicine cabinet. It can be used for treating a host of common problems including sore throats, thrush, nappy rash, sinus infections, athlete's foot and much more. 'Studies from a list of prestigious institutes have demonstrated grapefruit-seed extract to be effective against over twenty disease-causing bacteria, more than thirty fungi, and a host of single-cell parasites' (Alan Sachs, 1994). Dr Louis Parish, MD, an investigator for the US Department of Health and the FDA, who has treated many people with intestinal problems, including dysentery, believes that grapefruit-seed extract 'gives more symptomatic relief than any other treatment'.

It was discovered by a doctor and Einstein laureat physicist who specialized in finding natural remedies. He discovered that when he threw grapefruit seeds on to his compost heap they did not rot. The extract he made from the seeds may turn out to be the most benign antimicrobial discovered so far.

One of the disadvantages of conventional antibiotics is that they also kill off helpful bacteria, such as bifidobacteria and lactobacilli, in the gut. After treatment with Citricidal the bifidobacteria was unaffected and the lactobacilli only slightly reduced. Even more remarkably, this natural product also kills some viruses. William

Shannon of the Microvirology Division at the Southern Research Institute found it was effective against herpes simplex (cold sores) and one of the influenza viruses.

A South American laboratory, Interlab, has also found that Citricidal inactivated the measles virus, and the US Department of Agriculture found that it was effective against four animal viruses, including foot and mouth disease and African swine fever.

Other laboratory tests have shown that grapefruit-seed extract can kill many of the common pathogenic organisms including streptococci, staphylococci, salmonella, pseudomonas, giardia, lysteria, legionella, *Helicobacter pylori* and *Capylobacter jejuni*. Dr Leo Galland, who prescribes it for chronic candidiasis, has reported treatment failure in only two out of 297 cases, and considers it to be 'a major therapeutic breakthrough for patients with chronic parasitic and yeast infections . . .' (An information pack of laboratory test results, reports on the use of grapefruit-seed extract and a protocol sheet is available on request from Higher Nature – see Useful addresses.)

7

Allergy-induced headaches

Allergic reactions

These are a hypersensitivity to certain substances either inhaled, ingested, absorbed through the skin or manufactured in the body, for example, the toxins from invading bacteria or viruses. The immune system protects the body by trying to eliminate substances which it does not recognize (allergens), and an excessive reaction results in allergic symptoms such as swelling and overproduction of fluid. Common allergic reactions are seen in hay fever, asthma, eczema and nettle rash. These are well recognized, as are severe allergic reactions to one or two foods, and these have to be avoided throughout life, since they can produce severe breathing difficulties.

What happens during an allergic reaction?

A chemical called histamine released by the mast cells is over-produced and causes:

- dilation of blood vessels
- swelling in the linings of the airways – lungs and sinuses
- increased fluid at the site of injury
- increase in flow of tears and nasal secretions
- increased production of stomach acid
- itchy, inflamed skin.

The role of the immune system

The healthier the immune system, the more able it is to cope with allergens. If the immune system is depleted through ill health, stress, poor diet, lack of exercise or overuse of drugs, including alcohol, the development of allergic reactions is much more likely. Often people say, 'Why is this happening? I seem to be allergic to so many things at the moment.'

The production of antibodies

The production of antibodies by the immune system is vital to kill off invading micro-organisms or deal with certain substances. When an allergen is encountered for the first time, white blood cells known as lymphocytes are produced and attach themselves to other white blood cells known as mast cells. On the *second* encounter with the same substance the allergen binds to the antibodies on the mast cell, causing the release of chemicals called mediators which help to destroy the invader if it is a micro-organism. If it is a chemical the immune system cannot tolerate, an allergic reaction is the end result.

The importance of the second exposure

People with food intolerances need to understand that it is the second encounter with the allergen which causes the reaction. Hence, if you have become intolerant to wine and you have some at a dinner party you can feel fine but if you take it again the following day, even half a glass, you could have a reaction.

Food and chemical intolerance

This condition does not produce the dramatic symptoms of severe allergy, and is sometimes called masked or hidden allergy (see Mackarness, 1977). Food intolerance is an inflammatory response by the body to foods which are eaten regularly. When they are stopped, cravings and other withdrawal symptoms can develop. This has been much more frequent in the past thirty years, and could be the result of the human immune system not being able to cope with junk foods, or to an increase in prescribed drugs and environmental pollutants. The diagnosis is not well recognized and is often confused with other conditions, particularly psychological problems. This is possibly because there are many symptoms which are not clearly defined. It is often treated as hypochondriasis.

The allergy headache

Migraine can be triggered by certain foods and chemicals (p. 37); the offending substances seem to be the amine-rich foods such as cheese, chocolate or red wine (see p. 38), while those who suffer from food intolerances and hence headaches would be more likely to react to a much wider range of foods.

The typical allergy headache differs from migraine in that:

- the pain is not localized – it is an 'all-over headache';
- the pain is generally less severe;
- many of the accompanying symptoms do not appear in migraine attacks.

The sufferer often complains that the brain feels swollen, that they feel fuzzy or heavy-headed, they lose concentration and sometimes have feelings of unreality. Mood swings are also common and the sufferer can suddenly feel depressed and have a dull headache after eating an offending substance. Some people feel sleepy with this headache; others feel restless.

Symptoms which can accompany allergy headaches

- flushing, sweating after meals
- palpitations
- itchy, sore eyes
- bags or deep black shadows under eyes
- earache, itching in ears
- foul taste in mouth, loss of taste
- sore mouth, mouth ulcers
- swollen lips
- recurrent sore throat
- abnormal thirst
- stuffy nose
- sinus problems
- tight chest
- asthma
- hives (nettle rash)
- inflamed digestive tract
- bloating
- continuous dull abdominal ache
- colicky pains
- indigestion
- constipation
- diarrhoea
- flattened stool
- feeling of never having a complete bowel movement
- itching anus
- frequency of urine

- urgency of stool
- muscle or joint pain
- heavy legs
- feeling of the brain being swollen
- irritability, outburst of rage
- feeling of being 'spaced out'
- anxiety or depression after eating certain foods
- chronic fatigue
- hyperactivity.

Predisposing factors in food and chemical intolerance

- genetic influence
- stressed immune system
- environmental factors
- harmful bacteria, candida overgrowth (Trickett, 1994), parasites in the gut
- drugs
- inflammation in the gut (Trickett, 1990)
- damage to gut wall – 'leaky gut' (Trickett, 1990)
- lack of hydrochloric acid or enzymes
- disturbance of pancreatic function
- low levels of butyric acid made in the gut (see Neesby, 1990).

Allergic rhinitis headaches

Hay fever

Hay fever, caused by inhaling pollen, creates a vacuum headache: the blood vessels swell in the nasal passages and cut off the air supply to the sinuses. This tends to produce heavy or 'cotton-wool' headaches rather than severe localized pain. The eyes are itchy, red and swollen, and water profusely; the nose streams and is red and swollen. (The copious fluid is an attempt to wash away the offending pollen.) The throat is often red and scratchy. If the condition becomes chronic it can be complicated by infection. With hay fever, unlike other forms of rhinitis not due to pollen, symptoms disappear in the autumn and winter months. Homoeopathy can be an extremely effective treatment for hay fever, as it deals with the constitution as well as the distressing symptoms. Taking the strain off the immune system by omitting additives from the diet has helped some people (Freedman, 1977).

Other inhaled substances which may cause headaches

- dust mites
- animal hairs
- brake fluid on trains
- exhaust fumes
- printers' ink
- tobacco smoke
- gas, oil, factory fumes
- air fresheners
- formaldehyde
- fumes from chipboard furniture, synthetic carpets (the fumes from these decrease with time)
- chemical inhalants from plastics, adhesives
- flooring in shopping areas.

Chemical allergy headaches

These can be more severe than hay fever, probably because of toxins reaching the brain; profuse mucus production is not necessarily a feature.

Symptoms include:

- dull, throbbing, generalized headache
- restlessness
- mood swings
- inability to breathe through nose
- vague nausea
- swollen abdomen.

What to do

It is not always possible to exclude the substance affecting you from your environment. The first thing to do is to identify what substance is causing problems and if possible wear a protective mask, ventilate your working area and take frequent breaks in the fresh air. Work to build up your immune system (p. 54). As well as treating the symptoms, you must also build up your general health. See your doctor for referral to an allergy unit and possibly for a prescription for a non-sedative antihistamine, or look for a homoeopath.

Drugs for rhinitis

Drugs only suppress the symptoms – they do not cure the condition. They can also give you more troubles than you started with, so caution is necessary. If you cannot eliminate the substance from your environment in the long-term it is better if you can be desensitized.

Antihistamines

These are also known as H[1] blockers; they are the most widely used drugs in the treatment and prevention of allergies. They inhibit the activity of the mast cells and reduce the amount of histamine produced. Their most common use is in the treatment of hay fever or rhinitis from other causes, such as animal fur or dust, when it is impossible to avoid all contact with the allergen.

Older antihistamines such as Piriton (chlorpheniramine) have largely been replaced by newer ones, such as Seldane, Triludan and Boots antihistamine tablets (terfenedine), which are less sedating. It is important to note, however, that some users still report a sedative effect and care should be taken when driving, operating machinery or at other times when full concentration is needed. It is also important to follow the instructions carefully and not to take with grapefruit juice. Other preparations available are Hismanal and Pollon-Eze (astemizole).

Side-effects

Side-effects include dry mouth, blurred vision, weight gain and difficulty passing urine.

Take care! Antihistamines can increase the sedative effect of alcohol and of any drugs which have a depressant effect on the central nervous system, such as tranquillizers, sleeping pills and antidepressants. They can have the opposite effect in children and make them hyperactive.

Sodium cromoglycate

This is another mast-cell inhibitor which limits the production of histamine; it is also used to prevent asthma and allergic rhinitis. It should be started before the hay-fever season as it can take several weeks to be effective. Initially a local reaction (more sneezing) can occur but this passes off after a few days. This is the only reported side-effect except, very rarely, an asthma attack. The nasal spray

Resiston is available over the counter. Sodium cromoglycate can also be given in capsule form for food allergies.

Decongestants

These reduce swelling in the nose in rhinitis and dilate the air passages in asthma. When the delicate mucous membranes are irritated, the blood vessels enlarge and increased amounts of fluid are produced. The result is the production of more mucus, which can be a breeding ground for micro-organisms. Decongestants allow the mucus to drain more freely. There are risks associated with these drugs, so if your symptoms are not too severe try steam inhalations with or without menthol crystals, Oil of Olbas (available from any chemist), eucalyptus or tincture of benzoin (Friar's Balsam).

Common decongestant drugs

- *phenylpropanolamine*, available as Mucron, Sinutab and Triogesic (with paracetamol); these can have a mild diuretic effect and can reduce appetite
- *pseudoephidrine hydrochloride*, available as Sudafed
- *ephedrine nasal drops* – these are the safest nasal drops in this group (sympathomimetic drugs; see British National Formulary, 1994)
- *xylometazoline nasal drops*, available as Otrivine.

Note These nasal sprays should be used for a maximum of seven days to avoid any risk of rebound nasal congestion.

Side-effects

Drugs which contain ephedrine and pseudoephedrine taken orally stimulate the sympathetic nervous system and for this reason are more likely to cause increased heart-rate and trembling. People with heart and blood-pressure problems, over-active thyroid glands or anxiety states should avoid these drugs. They are also unsuitable for people on monoamine-oxidase inhibitors (MAOI antidepressants).

Rebound congestion

When decongestants are stopped after being abused or used for long periods there can be an overreaction in the tissues due to the dilation of the blood vessels. Very careful use and gradual withdrawal is essential with these drugs in order to avoid chronic damage to the nasal mucosa.

How decongestants are used

This can be by nasal drops or sprays (local or topical action), or by mouth as tablets. Topical use is safer since the drug is poorly absorbed.

Caution if you are on any medication check with your doctor or pharmacist before you buy any antihistamines, nasal decongestants or cold cure preparations.

Case history

Man of 30

I started getting hay fever when I was about ten years old. Life was a misery every summer. Five years ago I had my first attack of acute sinusitis. Life seemed just one round of either hay fever or sinus problems. I was worried about taking so many antibiotics and in spite of decongestants I felt blocked up most of the time and the headaches were getting me down. My girlfriend persuaded me to see her homoeopath. I have to admit I was sceptical at first. It was right in the middle of the hay-fever season. Within a week I had improved enough to make me want to continue with the treatment. I went for three months. I noticed a big difference when the cold weather came. It was the first winter for five years that I had not had repeated sinus infections. The following summer I had a mild bout of hay fever at the beginning of the season and went back for more treatment. I realize now I should have had treatment before the pollens started flying. I had very little trouble for the rest of that summer and have not had any problems since. The homoeopath also gave me a diet – no dairy produce and lots of vegetables and fruit. I think this helped too. I eat cheese from time to time now but I have kept off milk.

Other approaches to treating rhinitis

Allergy testing

Your doctor can refer you to the allergy department of an NHS hospital if you have respiratory symptoms (asthma, hay fever); the allergen causing the trouble can then be identified and treated by desensitization. Some hospitals also investigate and treat food intolerances.

If you find your doctor unwilling to accept your suspicions that food or chemical intolerance could be your problem, you may want to seek out a private clinic with a doctor who specializes in nutritional medicine. Other options are to find an alternative practitioner who is knowledgeable on the subject. (Many are.) If you have to rely on self-help, follow an elimination diet to find out what is affecting you. A colon cleansing programme plus nutritional supplements can help to build your immune system (Trickett, 1990). Chapter 12 deals with other ways of boosting the immune system.

The skin prick

In order to test for allergies, drops of liquid containing the common allergens are placed on the skin, which is then pricked or scratched. If the patient is sensitive to the substance, inflammation of the area – known as the weal-and-flare response – develops. This is a standard test for inhaled allergens such as pollens and dust, but is unreliable for food intolerances. Sublingual drops (drops placed under the tongue) are also used to identify allergens and they are used in dilute concentrations for desensitization treatment.

Intradermal injections

These are more reliable; they go deeper into the skin than the prick. If the person is not allergic to the substance a small weal which soon disappears is produced. In a positive reaction the weal increases in size and becomes white and hard.

Neutralization

This treatment is based on finding a dilution of the offending substance which will 'turn off' the allergic reaction by its influence on the immune system (see Mackarness, 1985). It is not known why neutralization therapy works, but it seems to have close parallels with the homoeopathic principle of like curing like – that is, the correct dilution of whatever the body considers a poison effecting a cure.

Enzyme-potentiated desensitization

A mixture of food extracts plus an enzyme is applied in a plastic cup to a scrach on the skin. Desensitization is presumably effected in the same way as in neutralization. This method of treatment is only needed about once every three months, and then less and less often as the immune system recovers. You are more likely to find this method in a private nutritional medicine clinic.

Kinesiology

Kinesiology or muscle testing is a simple and popular technique used by some doctors and many alternative therapists. It is based on muscle-testing techniques through which weaknesses are identified and treated. An antigen is placed on the surface of a patient's body (usually the abdomen), and certain muscles are tested for strengths and weaknesses. This is painless and effective, and the results are known immediately. Once the allergens are identified, homoeopathically prepared drops are administered, made from the offending substance, and this is usually given over a week, or two weeks if the allergy is persistent. These drops desensitize the patient and he/she is usually able to resume being in contact with the offender without any further problems. Usually one or two major allergens are found and once these are treated, the minor allergies usually clear up of their own accord. A full case history is taken before the testing begins.

Jane, a 29-year-old divorced woman with two children, complained of migraines which started when she was 23. She was getting them approximately twice per week and her work was being seriously affected. She brought with her small samples of food that she ate daily or nearly every day. She had stopped chocolate, cheese and red wine about three years previously but she still developed the migraines. I began to test her muscles for strengths and weaknesses. When I tested her with sugar and coffee, I noticed an immediate weakness in her muscle. She was amazed. She then had to avoid all sugars and coffee for a week while she took the desensitizing drops. After three weeks I re-tested her and found the weakness had disappeared. So, very slowly, she reintroduced sugars and coffee into her diet and there has been no recurrence of her migraines.

(Thank you to Hazel White-Cooper and R. S. Hom for the information on kinesiology. For further information contact Donald Harrison at the Institute of Allergy Therapists – see Useful addresses.)

Food allergy

Food intolerance: the major offenders

A study reported in the *Lancet* (Alun-Jones, 1982) showed that the main food allergens in adults were wheat, corn, dairy products, coffee, tea and citrus fruits. Infants are more likely to react to milk, soy and beef (Jenkins, 1984). Symptoms in older children are often due to milk products, too much sugar, junk foods, food colourings and additives.

Food rotation

The principle of this is a diet involving rotation and diversification of food. You are most likely to become intolerant of foods you have eaten all your life. Food rotation allows the immune system to recover, by not bombarding it with the same allergen every day. Some people react to so many foods that they could not possibly exclude them all because they would become malnourished, so they eat most things but only once in four days. The body seems to be able to cope with this and many people do well on it. It is tedious: it involves eating everything to do with the cow (dairy produce and beef) on one day and everything connected with sheep (lamb, lamb's liver, ewe's milk yogurt) on another day, and so on, and also a different grain, vegetable and fruit on every fourth day. This is a much sounder nutritional approach than eliminating several foods from your diet permanently, because, if you eat them daily, you can develop intolerances to new foods in the diet which do not initially cause a reaction. However, caution is needed, for long periods on very restricted diets can lead to vitamin and mineral deficiencies.

The effects of food and chemical intolerance on children

- failure to thrive
- vomiting

- diarrhoea
- constipation
- headaches

- mental dullness
- recurrent ear, nose and throat problems
- black circles under eyes
- itchy nose
- sleep disturbances

- hyperactivity
- aggression

- bed-wetting
- excessive thirst.

In an observational study (Kuvaeva, 1984), all cases of a group of children suffering from symptoms of food allergies showed evidence of deficiencies of lactobacillus and bifidobacterias combined with enterobacteriaeae (harmful bacteria) overgrowth.

8

Headaches caused by jaw problems

The temporo-mandibular or jaw joint is situated just in front of the opening in the ear. You can feel the movement if you press your finger firmly in front of your ear and move your jaw up and down. The muscles of this joint can be damaged by tension in the jaw, the joint being out of alignment, teeth-grinding or arthritis in the joint. The pain arises from stress in the muscles or joint, or from inflammation.

This problem is much commoner than you might think: an estimated 75 million people in the United States have TMJ problems (Gelb, 1983), and nine out of ten people with tension headaches also suffer from TMJ problems (Dick, 1990). TMJ problems are often overlooked or misdiagnosed.

The importance of the jaw joint

The jaw acts as a centre of body balance. When the jaw is in the correct position it allows the head to rest comfortably on the neck. If the lower jaw is forced out of place the head will be thrown out of balance and all the muscles supporting it will have to strain in order to keep it in position on the neck. We have seen earlier that tension in the neck muscles can send a message of tension to the whole body. It is not surprising, therefore, that the symptoms of a misaligned jaw go far beyond local pain.

The TMJ syndrome

The syndrome may involve the following symptoms:

- headaches which are usually unilateral and can be severe;
- waking up with a headache;
- pain in the joint itself, lower jaw, upper jaw, forehead, face, throat muscles, behind the eyes, in the temple, scalp, tongue, shoulders and neck;
- stiffness or numbness in face or scalp;

- sore eyes, sometimes with swelling;
- one eye higher than the other;
- mouth on affected side turned up;
- abnormal wear in teeth on one side;
- nocturnal teeth-grinding (bruxism);
- laborious chewing over meals or bolting meals without chewing with resulting digestive problems;
- leg shorter on affected side;
- swelling in face;
- grating or clicking in joint when chewing;
- pain in ear when chewing;
- feeling of pressure in ear or hissing, roaring or ringing noises;
- sensitivity to noise; easily startled by noise;
- restricted movement: difficulty opening mouth wide or moving jaw from left to right or back and forth;
- tingling in fingertips;
- recurrent sinus, ear, nose and throat infections.

How does the jaw become malpositioned?

Genetic influence

We are often built asymmetrically. For example, one leg can be shorter than the other and teeth may erupt irregularly. Since the teeth determine the position of the jaw, uneven teeth will not offer the full support that the jaw needs.

Nutrition and chewing habits

These are important not only for the developing teeth but also to maintain the necessary bite. Children who suck their thumbs or hang on to their dummies or bottles too long may push their teeth out of position. Others clench or grind their teeth during stress. Adults do this too.

Other causes

Injury to the head and jaw, and holding the jaw in tense attitudes such as 'setting the jaw' in anger or holding it tense when on the telephone. Most TMJ problems are muscle-contraction or tension induced.

67

Stress and the jaw

The jaw is often the focus for stress-related habits such as:

- jaw-jutting
- pencil-chewing, nail-biting, continual gum-chewing
- nocturnal teeth-grinding
- propping jaw on cupped hands
- poor posture.

These actions cause the muscles to go into spasm and circulation is impeded. This causes malnourished areas of tissue which become painful trigger spots.

Things to consider

- Did your headaches begin after dental treatment?
- Do your dentures fit well?
- Did you have your teeth straightened as a child?
- Are your headaches immune to drugs?
- Does prolonged chewing bring on a headache?
- Is there tenderness in the muscles around the jaw?
- Does your jaw veer to one side when you let it hang?
- Can you insert the first three knuckles of your fingers into your mouth when it is as wide open as possible?
- Have you got missing teeth?
- Is one eyebrow higher than the other?
- When you gently clench your teeth, does the pressure feel the same at both sides?
- If you make an imprint by biting into a thick slice of soft bread are the indentations shallower on one side than the other?

Become aware of your jaw

There is no need for the teeth to come together except when chewing or swallowing. Train yourself to place the tip of the tongue behind the front teeth. It is impossible to jaw-clench when the tongue is in this position. Be aware of how you are chewing – use both sides of your jaw. Notice what happens to your jaw when you are talking. Are you thrusting it out – does it tense up?

Treatment

Professional help

Pain from TMJ problems can only be relieved by the jaw being repositioned correctly, either by dental work or by an occlusal splint made by an orthodontist. This will correct your bite and allow the tense muscles to relax. This should have a dramatic effect on your headaches. Any other measure taken will be of limited value until the mechanics are corrected. Once the normal circulation to the head has been established you should have fewer sinus, ear, nose or throat infections.

What else can I do?

- Relax more!
- Treat the pain with analgesics.
- If you can, seek help from a cranial osteopath, osteopath, masseur, acupuncturist, shiatsu practitioner or other pain-relief technique.
- Massage the tight muscles regularly yourself.
- Learn which essential oils help pain.
- Learn which acupressure points help the pain.
- See which helps pain most – the application of warmth or cold. Boots and Body Shop have jelly packs which can be either heated or chilled.
- Do regular neck-stretching exercises.
- Support your chin when you yawn.
- Be aware of how you are holding your head.
- If you can afford it, have Alexander lessons (see Useful addresses).

TMJ syndrome and stress

The TMJ syndrome is generally associated with spasm in the muscles of mastication as a result of physical and/or psychological stressors (Henderikus, McGrath and Brooke, 1984). It would make sense, therefore, to include relaxation therapy in your treatment even if you have been given an occlusal splint (see above). Many people who have had stress management as their only treatment have done well.

Case histories

Man of 37

It was my osteopath who referred me to the dental unit. I am very glad he did. I was given a split to wear at night and if I felt tense. It worked like magic: the headaches vanished. I wish I had known about these splints years ago. It has made such a difference to my life. I don't wear it all the time now; only when I am under pressure.

Woman of 29

I had spent years changing my diet, doing yoga and hunting for something that would help my migraine attacks, but nothing seemed to work. I saw a piece in a migraine newsletter on TMJ as a precipitating factor in migraine. It made sense to me. My brother (another migraine sufferer) and I had both had our teeth in braces for years when we were kids. I went rushing off hopefully to the doctor to be referred to a consultant but he said he thought it an unlikely cause of migraine and just gave me some painkillers. My dentist was more helpful. He pressed inside my mouth and around my jaw and neck and said he thought there was inflammation in the muscles and it would do no harm to have it checked, although he also said it might not be the cause of the migraine. He referred me to an orthodontist who said I did have a problem jaw and he could not understand why I had left it so long. He made me an occlusion splint and it has helped emormously. I still get the odd migraine attack but they are a shadow of what they were.

Just how effective are occlusal splints?
(From Factsheet No. 4, Migraine Trust)

Since the early 1980s there have been fairly frequent claims of the efficacy of certain dental treatments, usually in relation to alterations of the 'bite' for the treatment of migraine. Claims of success, including one bold statement that 90 per cent of migraineurs need not suffer, have been met with scepticism in many quarters, not least the dental profession itself. There was a dearth of results from properly controlled research and most of the claims were based on hearsay, or 'clinical experience'. However, in the late 1980s a few results appeared in refereed journals. The oral medicine department of Glasgow Dental School in which I worked has a large group of patients, some of whom seemed to have experienced marked improvement following the provision of a small plastic appliance or splint. The device covered either the upper or lower teeth, was only worn at night and appeared to work best in those whose attacks of headache started on waking from sleep or soon afterwards. The appliance or 'splint' separates the teeth, and in theory allows the jaws to find the most comfortable position. It may also prevent habits such as tooth-grinding or clenching which can act as headache triggers (although not necessarily for migraine).

This experience suggested that there was some benefit to migraineurs which, if it was targeted correctly, could improve the quality of life of quite a lot of people. However, the complexity of individual migraine histories meant that it was difficult to be sure whether the reduction was in actual migraine attacks, or other headache types, for example tension headaches which were occurring in combination. The problem of a 'placebo-effect' of splint wearing must also be addressed.

With the help of a grant from the Migraine Trust, I was able to set up a clinical trial to investigate the potential benefits of splint wearing. About forty people who had been diagnosed as migraineurs by their general practitioners or neurologists were selected to take part. To take part in the trial all the participants had to experience attacks frequently (at least twice a month) and to report at least half of their attacks to begin on waking or soon afterwards. As the splint was only for night wear, it was important to target those whose attacks were triggered during the night, and this was the group who had previously been reported as most likely to benefit. At this stage the accuracy of the original diagnosis was not particularly important as each attack was to be diagnosed objectively during the trial.

All of the participants recorded the details of each attack on a separate form for a ten-week spell before treatment, and were then given an active splint or a placebo splint (which did not cover the teeth) on a random basis for another ten-week period. Those who wore the placebo were given an active splint to wear for a further period of ten weeks. During all of this time the patients recorded the details of every attack, which made a diagnosis possible for each one. All the forms were then analysed blind and a diagnosis of each attack was made, by rigidly applying the most recent diagnostic criteria, and its duration calculated.

The results produced some interesting findings. Firstly, many of those who suffered from migraine attacks also suffered from tension headaches. About a quarter of the patients who completed the trial showed a measurable benefit; in some cases it was very marked, but the biggest reduction tended to occur in those who suffered frequent tension-type headaches. Where both tension-type headaches and migraines occurred together it was the tension attacks which usually showed most reduction. Statistical analysis suggested that attacks of migraine with aura (classical migraine) were unaffected. Migraine without aura (common migraine) appeared to be reduced but the reduction was only slightly greater than would be expected by chance, and even using the available diagnostic criteria separating these from tension headaches is not always easy. Tension headaches on the other hand showed a marked reduction, in some quite dramatic. Two patients who had suffered almost daily headaches saw them almost completely eliminated.

Unfortunately the original promises of a wonder cure for migraine do not seem to hold. The successes in treating migraine in the past may have been due to the elimination of more frequent tension headaches which were occurring alongside attacks of migraine. However, we should not underestimate the benefits of this treatment. Many migraineurs' lives are made even more miserable by frequent, wearing, tension headaches, which occur in addition to their attacks of migraine. For a proportion of these people, particularly those who often wake up with headaches, an occlusal split may provide some relief.

J. G. Steele
Newcastle Dental School

9

Low blood sugar and headaches

What is hypoglycaemia or low blood sugar?

The food we eat is processed and enters the circulation as a form of sugar. By this route all cells receive the fuel necessary for normal functioning. The pancreas secretes the insulin necessary to metabolize carbohydrate, and unless there is diabetes or, less commonly, an inherited tendency to have faulty carbohydrate metabolism, this system works well. Careless eating habits, high levels of anxiety and taking or withdrawing from certain medications can also give rise to hypoglycaemic symptoms. There are three types of hypoglycaemia: reactive, diabetic and organic.

Reactive hypoglycaemia

Reactive hypoglycaemia is by far the most common type. It is what it suggests: the body is reacting to the way it is being treated. The pancreas is being overtaxed by a high sugar/refined carbohydrate diet, missed or late meals, alcohol, caffeine, nicotine and other drugs (mentioned later), or stress. This type of hypoglycaemia responds to self-help methods such as diet and stress reduction.

Some foods, irrespective of their carboyhydrate content, can produce an abnormally high or low blood sugar if the person is intolerant to them (Davies and Stewart, 1987). If your symptoms do not respond to the hypoglycaemic eating plan (see below), then you would do well to investigate food intolerances. You could start by cutting out the main allergens: wheat, dairy products and citrus fruit.

Diabetic hypoglycaemia

When a diabetic takes too much insulin the result is a dramatic drop in the blood sugar level.

Organic hypoglycaemia

This can be the result of an over- or under-active thyroid and would need to be investigated by your doctor. It can also occur after a partial gastrectomy. A rarer cause is organic disease of the pancreas or liver.

Diabetes

This condition develops when the pancreas fails to secrete enough insulin to cope with the carbohydrate it is presented with. The result is that the sugar cannot be broken down and used by the body. The blood sugar levels become too high, *hyper*glycaemia, and sugar is excreted in the urine. Without treatment the sufferer would quickly become dramatically ill. Treatment consists of insulin injections/drugs and a diet with a measured daily amount of carbohydrate to meet the energy needs of the person. If the diabetic is given too much insulin or if he fails to eat the required amount, his blood sugar level drops and he becomes *hypo*glycaemic.

Many doctors believe that low blood sugar symptoms are of importance only in diabetics. Others, particularly those who work in nutritional medicine, believe that hypoglycaemia is a much neglected condition responsible for many of the chronic health problems which plague modern man. The digestive system in man is built for the slow absorption of complex carbohydrates, such as whole grains, vegetables, fruit, protein and fat. This gives the body a steady supply of glucose during the day and enough to last through the night during rest. The quick sugar fixes of the modern diet cannot do this. The constantly overworked pancreas produces an excess of insulin and the body reacts with a multitude of symptoms.

When the blood sugar levels are low

Symptoms

- fatigue
- irritability
- headaches
- migraine
- dizziness
- fainting
- blurred vision
- twitching of muscles around the eye
- poor concentration
- forgetfulness
- anxiety
- panic attacks
- phobias

- depression
- wakefulness
- waking between 2.30–4.30 a.m.
- feeling of inner shaking
- cold hands and feet
- numbness
- joint and muscle stiffness
- little desire for breakfast
- food cravings, particularly sweet foods or drinks
- alcohol craving
- excessive smoking
- allergies
- epilepsy in susceptible individuals.

This is an awesome list of symptoms. It could be questioned whether it is possible for such a multitude of ills to stem merely from hypoglycaemia caused by careless eating habits or by an exhausted nervous system. However, the disappearance of these symptoms, many of which might have been very long term and resistant to all other treatments, in people who have adhered to the diet given below, cannot be questioned. For full explanations of why these symptoms develop, see Budd, 1981.

The above symptoms appear in other conditions, particularly nervous problems. Anxiety may be characterized by:

- sweating
- palpitations
- trembling
- headaches
- digestive upsets
- changes in appetite
- blood sugar problems
- urinary problems
- skin problems
- neck and shoulder tension
- dizziness
- ringing in the ears
- blurred vision
- sinus problems
- backache
- wobbly legs
- insomnia
- waking around 5 a.m.
- irritability
- confusion
- restlessness
- hopelessness
- hyperactivity
- lack of concentration
- rapid speech
- rapid thoughts
- paranoia
- phobias
- feelings of gloom and doom
- morbid thoughts
- crying easily
- laughing inappropriately

- tight chest
- overbreathing
- difficulty swallowing
- loss of interest in sex

- fainting
- attention seeking
- suicidal thoughts.

It is not surprising that there are many common symptoms in these two lists, and it is also understandable that both lists are so long. If the nervous system is under strain every system in the body is affected, whether the cause is worry or low blood sugar problems. People often ask why they get dramatic psychological symptoms (mood swings, panic, depression) if they skip meals, when they can still function physically: 'I'm not normally a nervous person.' The answer is that the muscles can utilize fat and protein to keep going in the absence of sugar, but the brain cannot. It relies entirely on a form of sugar to function, so confusion, headaches and so on are often the first symptoms of hypoglycaemia to appear.

It would be unwise, however, to assume your problems are necessarily due to hypoglycaemia. No matter how closely you identify with the list of symptoms, since many of the same symptoms appear in other conditions a medical check-up is necessary. If, on the other hand, you have seen a doctor and he maintains that it's just your nerves, you could still be greatly helped by following the diet principles described below.

Is it an illness?

Hypoglycaemia is not an illness but merely a reversible state. The treatment consists simply in changing the diet – if the symptoms, headaches, panic attacks, and so on disappear with careful eating, they are due to hypoglycaemia; if they don't, they are not. The following is taken from my book *Coping Successfully with Panic Attacks* (Trickett, 1992):

I have seen hypoglycaemia in a clinical setting on a diabetic ward and also in the community when working with people with anxiety and addiction problems. In the latter groups, perhaps the condition could more accurately be called unstable blood sugar levels rather than low blood sugar levels because symptoms can occur when the blood sugar levels are within normal limits. It would appear that it is sudden drops which cause the problems rather than the blood sugar level being abnormally low. It is interesting to note that blood taken whilst patients were actually having panic attacks was on the lower end of the scale but never actually below normal, and yet their symptoms responded very dramatically to a diet designed to keep the blood sugar levels stable.

After seeing hundreds of people improve, here and in America, when following a low blood sugar eating plan (which needs to be a lot more than just sensible eating), I feel it has a huge part to play in the management not only of anxiety, but also of migraine, PMT and some types of asthma.

Whilst I see it as an important part of treatment, I also feel strongly that the approach to it should be one of common sense. In the absence of organic disease, glucose-tolerance tests are not only a waste of time, but can also make the patient feel very unwell for several days.

I see the answer as very simple: if the symptoms are coming from unstable blood sugar levels, they will begin to respond to diet within a few days. If the patient has not seem a dramatic improvement within three months, then it is not a blood sugar problem.

In my work in the community over the past twelve years, it has been a great joy to see so many 'no breakfast, sandwich lunch, large evening meal' eaters reduce their adrenalin levels, lose so many of their headaches and anxiety symptoms, and become confident and in charge by simply stopping their blood sugar levels from kangarooing.

Low blood sugar – shall I go to the doctor?

Unless you feel you have developed low blood sugar symptoms since you have been on a prescribed drug it is probably a waste of time to go to your doctor. My experience of the general medical reaction to this problem is: 'Yes, it is hypoglycaemia – drink sweet tea!' or 'No, only diabetics get that when they have too much insulin; you are just anxious.'

I quote now from my letter to the *Relaxation for Living Newsletter*. This was written in response to the profession being worried about lay people using the term hypoglycaemia. There was also some denial that the control of low blood sugar levels was an appropriate part of anxiety management. I was puzzled by this because I feel that it is necessary to explore all avenues by which the overproduction of adrenalin could be controlled.

We have seen that when the body is under stress the circulation is affected and the result is palpitations, missed heartbeats and so on. In addition to the expected anxiety symptoms there are some which are more specific to changing blood sugar levels. These are dull headaches, inner trembling but no visible shaking, sugar craving, waking between 2 a.m. and 4 a.m. alert, anxious and sometimes very hungry, low energy mid-morning and mid-afternoon, twitching eyelid muscles, wanting to eat again about an hour after an evening meal, no desire for breakfast, lapses in concentration, tenderness over the pancreas and sore trigger points over the left lower ribs.

Other conditions associated with unstable blood sugar levels

While many doctors believe that low blood sugar levels are just something you get if you read too many women's magazines, others take the condition very seriously, believing that there is a connection between long-term hypoglycaemia and the development of chronic problems such as:

- overweight
- hyperactivity
- anxiety
- depression
- asthma
- loss of interest in sex
- fainting
- blackouts
- facial pain
- epilepsy
- arthritis
- allergies
- migraine
- stomach ulcers
- addictions
- tinnitus.

Principles of eating to keep the blood sugar stable

Hunger

The first rule is never to allow yourself to become hungry. The brain responds to the message of hunger by releasing adrenalin to access the store of sugar in the liver. High adrenalin levels produce trembling, headaches and the symptoms which have already been discussed.

78

Dangers of modern eating habits

Saving calories until the evening meal and having a 'blow out', perhaps because of fear of becoming overweight, is harmful in several ways.

- Fuel is needed during the day when you are active and less in the evening when you are resting.
- If the blood sugar levels are unstable during the day, by the time the pancreas is presented with the evening meal it is already so jittery that it may overcompensate with too much insulin and therefore within an hour or a little more after the meal your blood sugar level can be *lower than before you ate!* This is the time when you reach for biscuits, etc. You will probably have already done this mid-morning and mid-afternoon.

Will I gain weight on a diet to stabilize blood sugar levels?

You should *lose* weight, for three reasons:

1 Insulin is often called the fat hormone. The more insulin you produce the more fat you are likely to lay down.
2 You will not be consuming the 'empty', that is non-nutritious, calories of sugar and refined carbohydrates. These are the danger foods as far as excess weight is concerned.
3 Your energy levels should rise considerably. This will make you more active and you should metabolize your food more efficiently.

What if I lose too much weight?

Simply increase the amount of complex carbohydrate, including potatoes, that you eat until your weight stabilizes. Also eat larger portions of allowed foods. Do not be tempted to revert completely to a high sugar diet, but perhaps you can be a little more flexible with dessert after your main meals.

What should I eat?

Carbohydrate

There are several approaches to eating plans to stabilize blood sugar levels. The one suggested on p. 81 is the most popular one. High whole-grain diets with or without meat, and the macrobiotic diet (see Kushi, 1985) can also be used.

Another approach is to restrict carbohydrate to two or three slices of wholemeal bread, or less, or the equivalent in crispbread such as Ryvita. Some of this ration could be eaten as a wholegrain cereal, for example porridge, for breakfast (add seeds or nuts). If you work hard physically you might need a little more. If you are sedentary and overweight you could probably manage on less. Many people panic at the thought of restricting carbohydrate. This is a very useful eating plan for the obese or those who have difficulty digesting grains. There is no need to. If you are eating plenty of the allowed foods you should not be hungry.

Vegetables

Eat as many as you wish, raw or cooked.

Fruit

Include fresh fruit and unsweetened fruit juice to the equivalent of four to five pieces of fruit per day. This might seem more than what is allowed in other low blood sugar diets but should not be a problem unless you need to lose a lot of weight. The sugar in fruit (fructose) does not need insulin for digestion and therefore should not overstimulate the pancreas. The fruit and juice intake should include a high quantity of apple. Apple pectin helps to stabilize blood sugar levels (Werbach, 1987). Bananas are higher in carbohydrate than other fruits and should be limited to one per day.

Protein

Many of the earlier hypoglycaemic diets were very high in protein, but this has been found to be unnecessary; normal helpings of animal or vegetable protein suffice. Protein is a vital part of this eating plan. If you do not eat protein with each main meal you will not stabilize your blood sugar levels and are much more likely to crave sweet foods.

Fat

Unless you have been advised by your doctor to eat a low fat diet, include a moderate amount of fat in the diet. The trend for very low fat diets could have contributed to the rise in hypoglycaemia. There are also other hazards. Women on low fat diets have been shown to have a higher incidence of depression and suicidal tendencies (Hyman, 1992). A meal which includes fat stays much longer in the stomach than a low fat meal. Some of the foods you will be including actually reduce the cholesterol levels. They include apples, onions, garlic, olive oil and unrefined oats. Oat bran also has the advantage of stabilizing blood sugar levels (Werbach, 1987).

Do not eat

Refined carbohydrates

All white flour products such as bread, biscuits, cakes, sweetened refined breakfast cereals and pastries are out.

Sugar

Sugar in all forms, confectionery, dried fruit, soft drinks, is out. Look for hidden sugar in any prepared foods. In fact anything that tastes sweet, unless it states it contains only artificial sweeteners. These can be taken in small quantities, particularly at first if you are craving sugar. Liberal use helps to prolong your desire for sweet foods. If you keep to a sensible eating plan any desire for sweet foods should go within a few weeks.

Suggested diet

Fashions come and go with regard to the diet best suited to control the symptoms of hypoglycaemia. I have always favoured diets that were fairly high in protein (incidentally it has been found that hyperactive children do better on high protein diets). The latest research suggests that the ratio of protein to carbohydrate is of prime importance. The work of Dr Elias Ilyia in America has found that a ratio of one part protein to seven parts carbohydrate is the most effective eating plan. Dr Andrew Wright (see Useful addresses) favours one and a half parts protein to two parts carbohydrate. More information on this diet will be available in a forthcoming book by Dr Wright.

Quick reference

- Don't skip meals.
- Eat the allowed foods at regular intervals.
- Always have protein in your meals, particularly breakfast.
- Make the overnight fast as short as possible; if you wake in the night have a snack containing protein or complex carbohydrate.

- Cut down or abstain from caffeine (Ashton, 1987), alcohol, cigarettes and street drugs.
- Never smoke or drink alcohol before a meal.
- Do not drink alcohol during the day (O'Keefe and Marks, 1977).
- Consider whether you are using too many 'over-the-counter' drugs.
- Check with your doctor to see if all the medication you are taking is necessary.
- Watch your stress levels.
- Adopt better breathing habits.
- Take graduated exercise.
- Avoid too many late nights.
- Take a course of the recommended supplements (unless this conflicts with advice from your doctor).
- Always carry a snack (seeds, nuts, fruit, whole-grain low-sugar bar) with you in case you get delayed.
- In an emergency buy potato crisps; if you can only find a chocolate bar choose one with nuts in it and follow it with a protein meal as soon as you can.
- Don't try to fit your eating plan around others – your diet is important, it is your medicine!

Hypoglycaemia and nutritional supplements

Chromium

Chromium is the keystone for the glucose tolerance factor known as GTF which is thought to play a central role in the balance of blood sugar levels. Even with a sensible diet it is difficult to get the 125 micrograms of daily chromium recommended (*North East Times*, 1989). Inorganic chromium is poorly absorbed; organic Bio-Chromium is available in health stores and should be taken as directed by the manufacturers or your practitioner. Some people feel better within a few weeks of starting supplementation but a course of three months is recommended.

Magnesium

In an experimental controlled study of magnesium supplementation, blood glucose of hypoglycaemics failed to drop below fasting levels during glucose-tolerance tests; 57 per cent felt better versus 25 per cent of subjects on placebo (*North East Times*, 1989).

A six-week trial of around 340 mg daily for six weeks is suggested, unless you develop diarrhoea with this dose. Magnesium acts as a laxative.

People who have had nutritionally unsound diets for some time or those who are run-down could also include the supplements suggested for alcohol withdrawal below.

Alcohol

The strong connection between hypoglycaemia and problem drinking cannot be denied. There is a wealth of scientific information on this subject. The symptoms of a hangover are, after all, hypoglycaemic symptoms. The person with an inherited tendency to hypoglycaemia is much more likely to have problems with alcohol for two reasons:

- The alcohol gives him/her the same fix as a high-sugar/junk-food diet.
- Alcohol makes the store of glucose in the liver less accessible and so the problem drinker is in a vicious circle. In reaching for alcohol to stop withdrawal symptoms (including those of hypoglycaemia) he/she is in turn reducing the supply of glucose which would help the symptoms. People with alcohol problems invariably have a history and/or family history of blood-sugar-related conditions, such as overweight, migraine, arthritis and so on.

The problem drinker is so often seen as a weak person who cannot cope with the problems of life, or is judged as being irresponsible and hedonistic. The fact is that alcohol craving can be the result of biochemical imbalances and, in spite of the enormous amount of research which supports this, it is usually disregarded in general medicine. Old-fashioned notions of pleasure-seeking behaviour and the need to apportion blame abound. Animal studies are interesting and show that alcohol craving has its origins in the body, particularly the brain, and not in the psyche.

Laboratory rats were divided into two groups. One group was provided with a high carbohydrate 'junk' diet, the other with a biologically ideal diet. Both groups were given a choice of water or alcohol to drink. Both groups with a high sugar diet turned to the alcohol for drink, while their better-fed neighbours drank only water. These animals were not under stress, resentful, depressed, unhappy or frustrated. They just turned willingly to alcohol when their diet was inadequate. Furthermore, they became reformed alcoholics when their diets were improved and their carbohydrate level reduced (Budd, 1981).

Giving up or cutting down on alcohol

What you do about your alcohol consumption will probably depend on the degree of your symptoms. When people fully understand what alcohol is doing to their blood sugar levels many are willing to abstain completely for a while. From others the cry is 'But does that mean I can never enjoy a drink again?' The answer is no. When the body is balanced and healthy it can stand the strain of moderate weekend drinking or a couple of glasses of wine with a meal. When the blood sugar levels are swinging and the nervous system is overstimulated even half a pint of lager can cause severe symptoms. Alcohol affects more than the blood sugar levels, and if you normally drink heavily it would certainly make sense to give your body a complete rest from it for about six months. If you have tried this before and it was hell, remember that you have more information now, and with the correct diet and supplements it should be a great deal easier. In fact a great many people have said they did not intend giving up drinking completely but the desire just went once they were established on the diet. Smokers will find the craving for nicotine diminishes too.

Giving up

- Do not attempt this until you have been on the diet or diet/supplements for at least four weeks, but if you could cut down to a level where you are still comfortable, do.
- After four weeks keep very strictly to the diet: eat as many raw vegetables and salads as you can, and if necessary increase fruit and have drink diluted with apple juice when you would normally drink alcohol. (In an experimental study (Werbach, 1987) 32 hypertensive patients ate 62 per cent of their calories as raw food for six months; 80 per cent of those who smoked or drank abstained spontaneously.)

84

- Do not be tempted to increase your tea, coffee, coke intake. (In an animal experimental study (Register, 1972) one group of rats was fed a junk-food diet, the other received a well-balanced nutritious diet. When given either caffeine or coffee *both* groups increased their alcohol intake. This is not surprising, since the caffeine would stimulate the production of insulin and the resultant hypoglycaemia would, in turn, make the rats turn to alcohol for their sugar fix.)
- Take gentle exercise and get as much rest as possible.
- Encourage detoxification.

Gradual withdrawal

- Start the diet and cut down to a third of your daily intake of alcohol.
- After four weeks cut down to one or two glasses of wine, a pint of beer or one measure of spirits daily in the evening.
- Exercise and encourage detoxification as above.

It might seem strange in the light of the earlier information on the vicious circle of alcohol and hypoglycaemia that immediate and complete abstinence is not recommended for all sufferers. The reason for this is that complete withdrawal can be an enormous strain; withdrawal symptoms, in addition to the headaches, panic attacks and so on that the severely hypoglycaemic person is already experiencing, would for some people be rather a lot to cope with. But in saying that, if you know you cannot open a bottle without finishing it, you would be foolish not to go for complete abstinence. Take heart, the end results will be well worth it.

Alcohol/hypoglycaemia and behaviour

Hypoglycaemia is taken much more seriously in America as a cause of ill health and behavioural problems than it is in the United Kingdom. Studies have shown violent offenders in institutions to be happier and less aggressive when given a nutritional regime designed to keep blood sugar levels stable. The treatment has also been used for drunken drivers (*San Jose Mercury News*, 1993):

Jail time for some drunken drivers hasn't stopped them from

again drinking and driving. Now, San Mateo County is trying a new approach – taking away their coffee and candy bars.

In what could become a model for the state, thirty convicted drunken drivers . . . will participate in a new programme aimed at curbing alcohol abuse.

The regimen? Eat three protein-rich meals a day – and reduce caffeine and sugar.

Nutritional supplements

There are three reasons why the long-term heavy drinker has many nutritional deficiencies:

1 alcohol inhibits absorption of essential vitamins and minerals;
2 the heavy drinker would rather drink than eat;
3 the hypoglycaemia hangover prevents eating breakfast and often lunch, and high carbohydrate foods are craved towards evening.

Supplements and a well-balanced diet not only correct the nutritional status, but *can also do a great deal to minimize withdrawal symptoms and prevent relapse.* If possible, see a doctor who specializes in nutritional medicine, a nutritionist. (For telephone counselling see Useful addresses: Nutrition Line.) There are also many alternative practitioners who are very knowledgeable on nutrition. Here are some suggestions for supplements you will find in your pharmacy or health food store.

Caution Don't think that because you are swallowing a few supplements you can be careless about your eating habits. A well-balanced diet must be the choice if your income will not stretch to cover both.

Vitamin B complex

Choose a yeast-free one with 50 mg of the main Bs. People coming off alcohol are often prone to fungal infections (Trickett, 1994). Headache sufferers often have a reaction to niacin B3 (a harmless flushing and prickling of the skin which usually subsides within half an hour) so look for a product containing another form of B3 called nicotinamide. This has the same beneficial effect. B complex will make your urine a strange colour but don't let this cause you concern. The B vitamins can be stimulating, so take these with your breakfast. If you cannot tolerate the full dose build it up slowly by taking it three times a day or taking part of the tablet daily.

Multi-mineral tablet

This should include: calcium, magnesium, selenium, zinc and chromium (see p. 82).

Evening primrose oil

This is an EFA or essential fatty acid; $\frac{1}{2}$–1 g three times daily has been suggested to reduce the symptoms of alcohol withdrawal (Horrobin, 1982). Some people get headaches when taking evening primrose oil. If you cannot tolerate it, fish oil capsules would also be helpful.

Vitamin C

You can buy this in powder form from your pharmacist. It helps to rid the body of the toxins from the alcohol. This is another vitamin that can stimulate, so take it early in the day. If you can build up to 3 g per day without getting 'wired' – over-stimulated – or having digestive upsets it can be very beneficial.

Caution Supplements should be regarded as a medicine and as such kept out of reach of children. They should be taken as a course until you are well and not, unless under medical supervision, as a lifelong medication.

Other causes of blood sugar problems

Caffeine

Caffeine is a powerful stimulant; it can be consumed in large quantities in coffee itself, and in tea, coke, chocolate and some headache medications. Caffeine pushes the adrenal glands to raise the blood sugar level and insulin levels have to increase to keep pace with this. It has a similar effect to sugar and in addition has addictive properties. When the blood sugar levels are severely disturbed a cup of coffee or strong tea could be enough to produce severe anxiety symptoms. When treating hypoglycaemia, it is wise to give up coffee (you won't be having coke or chocolate because of their sugar content), but a word of warning about withdrawal. Like any other drug some people are more affected by withdrawal than others. This depends on what is going on biochemically and is not just the longing for the taste of coffee. When some coffee drinkers (even people who just have one cup per day) abstain they can for a few days suffer severe headaches and nausea, and can feel depressed for a couple of weeks. This is really due to caffeine poisoning, known as the 'caffeine storm'. In the absence of ingested caffeine, the caffeine in the body is mobilized and causes problems until detoxification is complete. To avoid this, cut down slowly by mixing half of your regular coffee with decaffeinated and progress slowly until you are drinking all decaffeinated.

Cigarettes

Nicotine stimulates the adrenal glands to release glucose into the blood. This is why it acts as an appetite suppressant. Your desire for nicotine should decrease when you are established on the hypoglycaemic eating plan.

Prescribed drugs and blood sugar problems

If change of diet is the prime cause of low blood sugar problems in modern man, then the massive increase in the use of prescribed drugs must be the second. Medical evidence now clearly states that the contraceptive pill, steroids, tranquillizers and sleeping pills, beta blockers and some diuretics (water pills) affect glucose tolerance, cholesterol and triglyceride metabolism. This adverse reaction often goes unnoticed because it is not dramatic. The onset is insidious and often not associated with the drugs either by the doctor or the patient (Taylor, 1986). For information on how to withdraw safely from tranquillizers and sleeping pills see Trickett, 1998.

Non-prescribed drugs

Street drugs, including heroin, cocaine and cannabis, all affect blood sugar levels and so when withdrawing from them the same principles of diet and nutritional supplementation apply as for alcohol withdrawal (above).

Children and hypoglycaemia

The behaviour of pale, irritable children crying for sweets at the supermarket checkout after school is the responsibility of the parent, not the child. If the child was given a wholemeal sandwich or an apple and cheese as it came out of the school gates many of these scenes would not occur. Children expend a vast amount of energy at school and many do not have a sufficient food intake to keep their blood sugar levels stable until they get home for tea. Ensure:

- that your child has a protein breakfast.
- that you ask staff about the quantity of food the young child eats at lunchtime;
- that you provide bananas or an apple for mid-morning and mid-afternoon breaks;
- that you meet the child with a snack;
- that you provide a substantial snack for the older child who has activities such as swimming or dancing after school;
- that you don't make young children wait for a family meal at 6 p.m. or later; give them a meal earlier and a snack before bed.

Hypoglycaemic children are fretful children who sleep badly and succumb to infections readily. They are also more likely to suffer from frequent headaches, transient abdominal pain, tantrums, asthma, eczema, allergies and hyperactivity.

Case histories

I have written books on a variety of health problems and they all include a chapter on hypoglycaemia. I can justify this by the wonderful letters I get from people all over the world who say that simply by changing their eating habits they have changed their lives.

Woman of 47

I read the literature on hypoglycaemia and in spite of several family members having conditions which would put me in line for hypoglycaemia I still did not take it seriously – it all seemed too simple. I had been a headache sufferer for years and often had palpitations and cold sweats. The doctor said it was my nerves. It was the accidental changing of my eating habits that made me take a second look at the information.

I was sent on a residential course for a week. Because they were put in front of me I ate three meals a day. I had not eaten a cooked breakfast for years. It was a boring week but I did notice that I had more energy and slept better. I thought it was just the change of scene.

On return home I reverted to my usual eating pattern and was rewarded with my familiar symptoms!

I have kept strictly to the diet now for seven months and feel a different person. I put on six pounds at first but am now back to my normal weight.

Woman of 39

I had high levels of sugar in my urine when carrying my first child (my grandmother was diabetic and my mother asthmatic). I was given a series of glucose tolerance tests, all of which gave me severe headaches and the shakes. My husband said it was the fear of the needles that made me nervous but I knew it was not that. I have never been afraid of injections. (He is the one with the needle phobia!) I was diagnosed as pre-diabetic and told to keep my weight down to avoid maturity-onset diabetes. That was all the information I was given. The result was that for years I ate very litle all day and had a big evening meal. I had years of being very uncomfortable after this meal; restlessness, palpitations, hot and cold flushes, and sometimes an inexplicable feeling of doom. I also had difficulty getting off to sleep and would wake regularly at 3.20 a.m. I knew the symptoms were something to do with eating, so I suspected food allergies. This was the wrong path and I was as frustrated as ever when I tried elimination diets.

I became a frequent user of the health section in the library and it was there I found a book on panic attacks which mentioned hypoglycaemia – it was all there. I feel a totally different person since I have been on the diet and know when I have 'lapsed'. I usually pay the penalty the next day in the form of a headache or a hung-over feeling.

10

Headaches and changing hormone levels

Headaches frequently accompany the changing hormone levels of puberty, the premenstrual phase, the menopause and pregnancy, although in pregnancy, particularly in the later stages (possibly because hypoglycaemia is less likely at this time), a woman may for a time be relieved of the migrainous headaches she has suffered from for years.

Headaches in the premenstrual and menstrual phase

These fall into three groups:

1 those caused by swollen cells; they are characterized by constant pain in the cheek-bones and forehead extending over to the back of the head, and sometimes accompanied by a stuffy nose and difficult breathing;
2 tension headaches caused by the effect of changing hormone levels on mood;
3 migraines caused by hormonal influences on the blood vessels in the brain.

The premenstrual phase

This can be described as a set of symptoms which appears seven to ten days before menstruation and disappears during or after menstruation. For some women it is just a minor cyclical discomfort. For others, it is a dreaded, fearful illness which destroys their confidence in themselves and their fitness for motherhood, and often their relationships with their partners and their ability to hold down a job. The symptoms are due to physiological changes which include changes in brain chemistry; the sufferers are perfectly well at other times in the month and are not 'neurotic' or hysterical, as sadly they are often labelled. The symptoms include:

• fatigue
• headaches

- palpitations
- dizziness or fainting
- constipation
- fluid retention
- swollen abdomen, thighs, ankles, hands and face
- tender breasts
- tingling of the fingers (usually the little and adjacent finger)
- numbness in the hands and arms after sleeping
- clumsiness – particularly dropping things
- low backache
- muscle and joint pains
- disturbance of blood sugar levels
- food cravings, extreme hunger
- temporary food intolerance
- restlessness
- irritability
- hopelessness
- insomnia
- anxiety, phobias, panic attacks, depersonalization
- depression
- mood swings
- violent feelings, actual violence
- suicidal feelings, suicide attempts
- oily skin or acne.

Women who have conditions such as asthma often have a worsening of symptoms premenstrually (Davies and Stewart, 1987). This is not surprising, since asthma can be affected by changing blood sugar levels.

Regular comments from sufferers

'I am a totally different person one week in four.'

'Each time, I think I'm going mad.'

'I can't convince my doctor about how ill I feel. He just offers me antidepressants.'

'It's the only time I ever smack the children. The guilt destroys me.'

'I know I will lose my husband if I don't get some help.'

'I'm terrified by how aggressive I feel – it's just not me. I never feel like that at any other time.'

'I have to get my mother to come to stay every month. I'm so afraid I will do something stupid. I don't feel like this at any other time. She was frightened at first but now she understands.'

'I live in terror of my children being taken into care. During that week they are strangers to me. My husband says I'm just being ridiculous.'

'I feel like a lumbering elephant and keep bumping into things.'

'My whole body aches as if I had flu.'

'As soon as I start to pass more urine the relief is immediate; my mood lifts.'

'I feel as if my head is bursting before my period.'

What to do about PMT

- Look carefully at your diet. How does it differ from the suggested diet for low blood sugar problems?
- How much exercise are you getting? You must move if you want the lymphatic system to work properly. Brisk daily walking for half an hour *during the whole of the month* should help to prevent retention of fluid. A weekly workout or aerobics class is not enough – a helpful extra, but not enough in itself.
- Look at your lifestyle. Look ahead to the end of the month and plan to take it easier during that time.
- Bombard your partner with literature on PMT.
- Explain to the children *before* the event that sometimes you feel irritable and that it is not their fault. Appeal to them to help you on the days when you are feeling unwell. Get them to colour on the calendar the days when you know your fuse will be short.
- If there is any extra help around, ask for it. You cannot help being subject to your hormones.
- Don't be ashamed of how you feel – unless of course you are not willing to look at how you can help yourself.

Nutritional supplements and PMT

Many sufferers find that adjusting the diet and taking supplements either completely cures or alleviates their symptoms. There are sound physiological reasons for this.

Magnesium

Magnesium has been shown to increase progesterone levels in the premenstrual phase (Davies and Stewart, 1987) and also reduces the symptoms of reactive hypoglycaemia (low blood sugar), which for many women is a large part of the PMT syndrome.

Vitamin B6

This vitamin increases red-cell magnesium levels and also helps to prevent fluid retention. Prescribed diuretics often deplete magnesium levels and therefore compound the problem (Trimmer, 1987). The B vitamins should never be taken in isolation because they deplete the store of the other B vitamins. So if you are taking vitamin B6, it is necessary to take a small dose of B complex daily or a larger dose two or three times a week. During the premenstrual phase 100 mg B6 is necessary daily; 50 mg or less can be taken during the rest of the month.

Vitamin B2

A three-month double-blind study at the General Hospital of Luxembourg and Belgium found that taking 400 mg of vitamin B2 per day has been found to prevent migraines. Some 59 per cent of sufferers said their headache frequency had fallen by at least half. They also reported that headaches did not last as long, showing that B2 could, for some people, be as effective as drug treatment but with none of the side effects. This is certainly good news, but it would perhaps be wise to speak with a qualified nutritionist if you intend to take a B vitamin supplement on a daily basis. If the B vitamins are taken in isolation they often deplete the other B vitamins. A way around this would be to take a low dosage B complex (making sure that your total intake of B2 does not exceed a total of the recommended 400 mg dosage).

Paradoxically B complex gives some people headaches or makes them feel 'wired'. It can also cause insomnia. If this is your experience then perhaps a natural B supplement such as chlorella (available from New Nutrition – see Useful addresses) would seem more sensible, and try to include as many foods rich in vitamin B in your diet as possible.

Essential fatty acids

We need fat in various forms to maintain health, including linoleic and linolenic acids – the 'essential fatty acids'. They have to be taken in the diet because they cannot be manufactured by the body. Foods high in EFAs include sunflower seeds, fish, shellfish, fish liver oils, safflower seed oil, corn oil, lean meat, kidneys, liver, pulses and green vegetables. Evening primrose oil is a very rich source. Your doctor may prescribe this for PMT. Vitamins B6 and C, and zinc are necessary for the absorption of evening primrose oil. A combination of these, called Efamol, is available at most pharmacies. Some people are unable to utilize their dietary intake of EFAs and research has shown that many conditions such as PMT, cardiovascular problems, rheumatoid arthritis, eczema, hyperactivity in children, inflammatory conditions, dry eye and even multiple sclerosis and schizophrenia can be helped by supplementation (Graham, 1984).

If you want more information ring Nutrition Line or The Premenstrual Tension Advisory Service (see Useful addresses).

The contraceptive pill

If you feel the pill is giving you headaches read Ellen Grant's *The Bitter Pill – How Safe is the 'Perfect Contraceptive'?* (1985).

Hormone replacement therapy

Some women feel wonderful on HRT, others suffer headaches and feel bloated and depressed. A natural HRT treatment is boron, a substance found in green vegetables. Clinical trials have found this supplement (often combined with calcium) as useful as synthetic hormones for controlling menopausal symptoms. It is available in most health stores or from Nutrition Line (see Useful addresses). This organization can also give you details of an exciting new cream called Pro-gest, which is used for menopausal problems, including osteoporosis. It is made from wild yams. Many doctors are prescribing this and the results are impressive.

Stress

When the body is under constant stress, hormone levels can be affected (men too). The adrenal glands can become exhausted and cortisol levels can be raised. A reliable test for information on how your adrenal glands and other glands are coping is available from Higher Nature (see Useful addresses). It is a simple saliva test and full instructions are sent with the test kit. A doctor trained in clinical nutrition or nutritionist will have to interpret the results and advise you on the supplements necessary to bring your body into balance.

11

Headaches and other problems caused by hyperventilation

I have covered this subject more fully in my book *Coping Successfully with Panic Attacks* (Trickett, 1992). If any of the books mentioned are not in your local library, they will order them for you for a small charge.

Six to eleven per cent of patients seen in a doctor's surgery breathe in a manner that causes health problems. The symptoms produced are often misdiagnosed because most doctors only recognize the symptoms of overt hyperventilation and overlook the signs of chronic subtle hyperventilation (overbreathing).

In common with hypoglycaemia, hyperventilation (sometimes called collar-bone breathing) is often seen simply as a sign of anxiety. Overt hyperventilation, where the patient is panting, gasping for breath and in an agitated state, is well recognized, but chronic low-grade hyperventilation is often not immediately obvious. The chronic hyperventilator breathes shallowly and rapidly, usually more than 16 times per minute, using only the upper part of the chest. The breaths often vary in depth, with an occasional deep, sighing breath. Breathing in this way deprives the brain of carbon dioxide. Any experienced telephone counsellor will be familiar with this sound. This breathing contrasts with normal breathing, which uses the abdominal muscles and where there is very little upper chest movement; it is silent and gentle, with a resting breathing rate of about eight to 12 breaths per minute.

It is unlikely that headaches will be the symptom of hyperventilation that takes you to the doctor, because the headaches are not usually severe – rather more generalized, dull headaches with a 'spacy' feeling. If you are overbreathing to the extent of getting very tense, you may have tension headaches. Migraine can also be triggered by hyperventilation (Lumb, 1987)

First aid for symptoms of hyperventilation

To re-breathe the carbon dioxide you are losing, place a paper bag around the nose and mouth, drop your shoulders and relax in a chair or on the bed. If you puff and blow into the bag you will make the symptoms worse. Just sit there and imagine your breathing becoming slower and slower. Continue for at least ten minutes and, if possible, have a rest or relax with a book afterwards. Do this as many times as you wish during the day or night.

Why do people develop this breathing habit?

Hyperventilation is another mechanism which suppresses feeling. It acts in the same way as the tightening of the muscles – it keeps in our emotions. Stress is the major cause of hyperventilation; some others follow.

Emotional triggers

These include suppression of fear, sadness, grief, anger and frustration.

It is natural for the breathing rate to increase when we are in a fearful situation. This gives us the impetus to run or challenge. When we are in a chronically anxious state we are continually halfway to the emergency mode and our breathing matches that state. Breath-holding can be a feature of hyperventilation. This could be an unconscious attempt to slow down the metabolism and the over-production of adrenalin.

Physical triggers

The only positive thing which can be said about hyperventilation (unless we are in a flight-or-fight situation) is that it can help to control physical pain, particularly in the chest and back. Imagine breathing deeply with broken ribs. The danger lies in the fact that often long after the pain has gone the sufferer retains the habit of overbreathing.

Tight clothing, working for long periods in a cramped position, gas in the stomach or bowel pushing up on the diaphragm, a stuffy nose, excitement, compulsive talking or muscular tension can all cause overbreathing. It could also be that deficiency of the B vitamins and a poor nutritional state could be another factor. A high-sugar diet can also be a cause, so the symptoms of hypoglycaemia and hyperventilation can coexist.

Taking a deep breath after relaxing may be an unconscious trigger which starts a hyperventilation attack. For this reason I am wary of commercial relaxation tapes which instruct people to take deep breaths.

How does the body respond to hyperventilation?

When the full capacity of the lungs is not utilized the correct balance of oxygen and carbon dioxide in the blood cannot be maintained, and the result is an alteration in brain chemistry which can lead to uncomfortable and often bizarre symptoms.

Even if carbon dioxide levels do not fall enough to give rise to dramatic neurological symptoms, continually overbreathing can result in being continually tired and in a nervous state. Because the onset of these symptoms is insidious and the sufferer may have had them for many years, it is often difficult to convince the person with poor breathing habits that they are themselves creating the symptoms which are disrupting their lives. Just as in hypoglycaemia, where sudden changes in blood sugar levels can cause dramatic symptoms, with hyperventilation sudden changes in carbon dioxide levels can produce dizziness, panic and headaches. This is why some people are so afraid to let go in a relaxation class; a few deep breaths can rapidly give rise to symptoms.

Symptoms of overbreathing

- yawning (air hunger)
- light-headedness
- dizziness
- headaches and migraine
- anxiety
- panic attacks
- depression
- feelings of unreality
- sense of hopelessness
- poor memory
- agoraphobia
- other phobias
- palpitations

- shortage of breath: inability to take deep breaths, frequent sighing (80 per cent of patients who hyperventilate sigh)
- dry throat: clearing of throat, moistening of dry lips
- dry cough: due to water and heat loss from mucosal lining of airway
- stuffy nose: dryness, sores in the nose, sniffing, dry lips
- chest pain: either a sharp pain lasting seconds or minutes or a dull ache over the heart and around the breastbone and ribs. This is caused by the strain on the muscles and ligaments by breathing continually from the upper chest.

  Finger pressure around breastbone or ribs can often find very sore spots. There is also an inability to lie on the left side. The pain is not usually affected by breathing.

  It can occur after exercise. Pressure from gas in the stomach can also cause pain.

  Spasm in the coronary artery can cause severe pain and often people arrive at accident and emergency departments (sometimes several times a year) with this
- feeling of impending fainting: all ages
- actual fainting: more common in the young
- tingling: hands, feet and around mouth
- weakness: in all muscles
- numbness: anywhere in the body
- jelly legs: a feeling that the legs cannot support the body
- digestive disturbances: water brash, bloating, belching, wind in bowel, air swallowing, food intolerances, irritable bowel syndrome.
- muscle spasm: particularly in the neck and shoulders; claw-like spasm in the hands and feet
- speech difficulties: feeling of tongue being swollen
- hallucinations: only when symptoms are severe. Children sometimes take gulping breaths and spin each other round in order to see 'pictures'
- increase in the effect of alcohol
- allergies: histamine production is increased by hyperventilation. Hyperventilators frequently exhibit food intolerances and have irritable bowel symptoms (Lumb, 1987).

Caution Hyperventilation can mimic many organic diseases. Consult your doctor if you have any of the above symptoms. If he/she can find no organic cause for your symptoms (they are far more likely to say you have nervous trouble than to notice your breathing), don't worry – get started on the exercises given below.

> Several factors foster the neglect of hyperventilation as a positive diagnosis, e.g. the absence of conspicuous overbreathing. Shortness of breath is seldom the primary complaint. But most important is the too-ready acceptance of the blanket diagnosis of 'neurosis' or 'anxiety state' to cover the inability of physicians to explain multiple symptoms without overt pathology (Lumb, 1981).

Headaches and hyperventilation

These are generalized, accompanied by a 'spacy' feeling and are not usually severe.

How do I know if I am hyperventilating?

If you have not identified with several of the symptoms in the above list your breathing patterns may not be a problem. For an additional check, count how many times you breathe per minute when you are at rest. If you feel anxious about this, however, your breathing will automatically speed up, so you might prefer to ask a friend to observe your breathing rate when you are not aware of what he/she is doing. The rise and fall of the chest count as one respiration. To calculate your breathing rate, look at a clock or watch with a second hand when you have been at rest for about ten minutes, count your respirations for 30 seconds and double this number; this will give you your breathing rate per minute. If it is 16 or more you would be wise to start breathing retraining. Some people try to rush this and complain of feeling breathless and panicky. If you attempt to go from rapid shallow breathing to deep breaths you *will* feel odd. If you have been breathing rapidly and shallowly for years, then it is going to take time to correct this, but with patience, just as your present breathing pattern has become habit, so will the fuller, slower breaths which will nourish all the cells of your body and calm your nervous system.

What to do

Initially you should forget about how you are breathing and concentrate on expanding your chest cavity. If your shoulders are held high, and your ribs and abdomen tense, they must be constricting your lungs. You cannot expect your lungs to work efficiently under these conditions. It's rather like trying to inflate a balloon in a cereal box!

The muscles

1 Lie down or relax in a chair with your head supported.

2 Drop your shoulders.

3 Put your hands on your abdomen and push them up towards the ceiling with your abdomen – relax, and then repeat twice more. Think about the muscles, not your breathing, as you do this.

4 Place your hands, fingers pointing to the centre, on your ribs. Push the ribs out to the sides as far as you can. There should now be a gap between your hands. Relax and repeat twice.

5 Pull your shoulders up towards your ears and then release them and push your hands down your thighs as far as you can. Repeat twice more.

Do not rush any of these exercises. Relax as much as you need to between them. Notice the feelings in your shoulders after you have let them go and don't be surprised if your gut rumbles – it has just been released from prison.

The breath

As you move around in your normal activity, avoid holding your shoulders around your ears and attempt to slow down your breathing *gradually*; making the out-breath longer than the in-breath will be a good start – remember, at this stage it is slow breathing, not deep breathing, you are aiming for. If you can do the following exercise twice daily and be vigilant about slowing your breathing at all times, the old habits will gradually fade. Don't expect miracles overnight – it has taken time to establish your present breathing habits and it will take time to correct them.

Relaxation using the complete breath

1 Massage under the instep of each foot firmly in a circular motion.

2 Lie down on the floor or bed with the head slightly raised. If you have back trouble, bend your knees and put your feet flat on the floor. If it is an effort to get up and down, relax in a chair with the head supported. Have a blanket near you. Initially relaxation can promote warmth but some people become very cold as deep tensions leave the body.

3 Choose a colour. Blue or green are the most sedating colours but you might prefer another. Imagine you are breathing this colour up through the soles of your feet, and it is going to gently lift your abdomen, ease out your ribs, go up into your shoulders and neck and out of the top of your head. Let it then cascade like a glittering fountain down over your body and over your feet. This must be done gently and rhythmically, like a slow wave washing up and over you.

4 Imagine the glow from this colour spreading to an area of about five feet around your body.

If you can, do this twice daily (on waking and before your evening meal, if possible) for ten minutes initially. Many people find the exercise boring and difficult at first but with patience you will soon enjoy the feeling so much that you want to extend the time – the longer you do it the more relaxed you will feel. Some people like to play music during their breathing exercises. If you get in a muddle just take a rest and start again.

What else can I do to help my breathing?

You can try graduated exercise, even simple stretching movements in the house, building up to brisk walking, swimming and, with your doctor's approval, aerobic exercise. Yoga is very helpful since it incorporates stretching and breathing exercises.

Are there breathing retraining clinics in the NHS?

There are a few hospitals where physiotherapists work with people to retrain their breathing, but unfortunately, unless you are severely agoraphobic or are overtly hyperventilating, it is unlikely that you would be referred.

Alternative therapies

Many alternative therapies can help hyperventilators. They include shiatsu, remedial massage and yoga.

Excerpts from sufferers' letters

I endorse what you say about hyperventilation in your book on panic attacks. Several years ago I was severely agoraphobic and generally very nervous. After a six-week breathing retraining course at Papworth Hospital I felt like a completely new person. I continued the treatment at home and within four months was able to go alone to the local shops. I am now totally free of nervous troubles and travel all over.

I refused to believe I was overbreathing and that my breathing could have anything to do with how I felt until my therapist asked me to visualize driving over a bridge (my worst fear). As I did this, although I was not aware of my breathing speeding up, all the familiar feelings of panic, tingling fingers and dizziness came. I found the exercises a bit tedious at first and it took me several weeks to really let go but I have to admit I feel much more in control and I have lost all those strange physical feelings.

I have never had a panic attack but what I called my 'queer heads', shortness of breath and digestive problems have gone since I learned how to breathe from my abdomen.

12

Paying attention to general health

The bowel

This might seem like an odd place to start when looking at measures to improve the general health. Perhaps most people would expect the accent to be on exercise and fresh air, with a footnote at the end reminding the reader to avoid constipation. When you understand that the bowel is not just a waste-disposal system but a vital part of your immune system, and learn how it plays a large part in determining your nutritional status, you might be more interested in learning how to keep it healthy.

A sluggish colon produces putrefaction. It was formerly thought that toxins from the colon could not enter the bloodstream; this is now known to be incorrect. Sufferers from the 'leaky gut syndrome' often get headaches.

What is a toxic colon?

'Toxic colon' is the term for a bowel which is carrying old faeces. It is not only a major factor in the development of the irritable bowel syndrome, food intolerances and chronic vague ill health, but it can also cause degenerative disease such as arthritis and cancer. You cannot expect to be well if the main organ responsible for ridding the body of toxic waste is underfunctioning. When the colon is irritated by diet, stress, drugs, chemicals and so on, it tries to protect itself by producing more mucus; this can bind with the sludge from refined foods, such as white flour, and build up on the wall of the bowel and narrow the passage. This layer of gluey, hardened faeces (which can weigh 3–4 kg and account for many distended abdomens) is not only an excellent breeding ground for harmful organisms, but also prevents the production of enzymes necessary for digestion, inhibits the production of vitamins and hinders absorption of essential vitamins and minerals taken in the diet.

Once a day?

Do not think that, because you have regular bowel movements or even diarrhoea, you have escaped this problem. The stool can pass daily through a dirty colon and leave the accumulated residue on the walls behind. There is no need to get panicky about this, as there is a great deal that can be done about it.

How does a toxic colon affect the body?

The local effects of this poisonous residue are irritation and inflammation. The general effects include diarrhoea, constipation, fatigue, headaches, dull eyes, poor skin, spots, aching muscles, joint pains and depression. The poisons circulate via the blood through a network of vessels called the lymphatic system to all parts of the body. Healthy lymphatic fluid should serve to nourish cells not fed by blood vessels; the lymphatic fluid also kills off harmful organisms and carries away the refuse. If the body has to pump around excessive toxic waste long-term it is not surprising that it sometimes has to give up and the disease process takes over: irritable bowel syndrome, colitis (inflammation of the colon), Crohn's disease (inflammation of the small intestine), colon cancer and diverticulitis.

Keeping the colon clean

The benefits of colon cleansing are manifold, not only in terms of health but also with regard to appearance: the skin looks vibrant, cellulite, water retention and blemishes disappear and the whites of the eyes regain a youthful clearness. How quickly you want to clean out is your choice.

What to do

Changing to a clean diet over a period of several weeks is described in my book *The Irritable Bowel Syndrome and Diverticulosis* (Trickett, 1990). If you also want to lose weight, two books on clean eating with a common-sense approach are *The Wright Diet* by Celia Wright (1986), and *Fit for Life* by Harvey and Marilyn Diamond (1987).

Cleansing the Colon by Brian Wright (available from New Nutrition – see Useful addresses) is an excellent booklet which describes how you can achieve a complete colon cleanse by diet, natural supplements and herbs.

Colonic irrigation

This practice had some bad press years ago because obsessive dieters abused it, but three or four treatments can be of tremendous value to remove an accumulation of old faeces. Most people think of this as some nightmare experience. It is far from this and there are many trained practitioners around the country using sterile up-to-date equipment. Some people feel lighter, and lose headaches, aches and pains, and other chronic symptoms after the first treatment. It is a swift method of cleansing the colon and it also obviates many of the unpleasant symptoms of detoxification. A sterile tube is inserted into the rectum and filtered water washes around the colon. It leaves via an evacuation tube, taking with it the accumulated debris and mucus of years. If you want to find a practitioner in your area write to the Colonic International Association (see Useful addresses).

The spine

A rigid or stiff spine causes not only local pain but can also affect the internal organs. Osteopaths and chiropractors believe that a flexible, straight spine is essential for a healthy body. Slight displacements of the vertebrae (called subluxations) interfere with the nerve supply, cause the surrounding muscles to go into spasm and can also be the cause of organic problems. Subluxation in the mid-thoracic region will not only cause discomfort between the shoulders but can also be the cause of digestive problems. Problems with the cervical spine often cause headaches and migraine.

It is a strain for man to be upright all day and support the head, which comprises quite a large portion of the body weight. A few simple stretching exercises daily could save you a lot of back problems.

The muscles

If you have ever compared the size of calf or forearm muscles which have been encased in plaster following an injury, to the size of the muscles on the uninjured side you will understand how not using muscles causes them to become flaccid and weak. To a lesser extent this is just what happens to all muscles when you sit in a car, behind a desk or in meetings for most of your day. We have seen how the systems of the body are interdependent: when the muscles are not used the waste products of metabolism are trapped, and aching and stiffness result; the circulation is slowed down, causing poor peripheral circulation and sluggish internal organs. If the lymphatic system cannot perform its task efficiently, the immune system suffers. Mood is also affected by lack of exercise: the more tense and tired the muscles are, the more the brain chemistry is affected. If the production of endorphins is low, then the mood will be low. The opposite of this is the 'runner's high'. You do not need to go as far as that, but don't be surprised if you are lethargic and mentally weary if you spend your time moving from car to office desk to a chair in front of the television set.

How much do I move my body each day?

Even if you have little time for planned exercise, you can build simple stretching movements into your daily routine by stretching your calf muscles as you walk upstairs, avoiding lifts and escalators; taking a brisk walk in your lunch break; rotating your shoulders while waiting for the kettle to boil; making a habit of doing a few stretching exercises before your shower.

This might all sound very tame but at least it is a start; it might also make you aware of how much your body needs exercise. At least it is better than doing nothing and better than a frenetic visit to an exercise class which makes you stiff and sore and discourages you from going again.

The skin

Since it is the largest excretory organ of the body, encouraging detoxification by skin brushing or water therapies is an important part of getting fitter.

Skin brushing

If you brush all over with a dry skin brush (available from Boots and New Nutrition – see Useful addresses) for about ten minutes before your bath or shower you will greatly stimulate your circulation, help the release of toxins and improve the texture of your skin. Avoid tender or broken skin, moles and pimples. After a few days you will notice how the normally roughened areas such as knees, feet and elbows become smoother and softer.

Improving your general health

Water therapy

The healing properties of water have been known for thousands of years. Even simple things such as stamping in cold water in the bath (for safety use a rubber bath mat) for three to five minutes or, better still, walking at the edge of the sea massages the soles of the feet and stimulates the hypothalamus gland. This increases the metabolic rate and produces a feeling of well-being. Pouring cold water after a warm bath (either from a shower or jug) down the spine can also produce this effect.

'Getting into hot water'

The profuse sweating of a fever is nature's way of detoxifying the body. You can do this artificially in Turkish baths and saunas, or at home in salt or Epsom salts (magnesium) or seaweed baths. These are all available from most pharmacists in large packs. A rough guide is to use about 2 lb of salt, three cupfuls of Epsom salts or one cupful of seaweed in a warm bath. The latter must be mixed to a paste in cold water and added gradually. Wrap up in a warm towel and rest for half an hour after your bath. Saunas and jacuzzis are also helpful for detoxification and relaxation.

Swimming

Regular swimming can help your mind as well as your muscles, but remember that doing the breaststroke, particularly with your face out of the water, can cause tension in the neck and shoulder muscles and this often results in headaches, pain in the neck and shoulders, and also backache. Water exercises are just as useful as swimming: walking or jogging back and forth across the pool; rotating the shoulders backwards underwater; pushing the arms from side to side underwater or holding on to the side and working with one leg at a time, rotating ankle, knee and hip joints, and then kicking the legs as far forward and backward as possible.

Fresh air

Filling the lungs with clean air has a tonic effect on the whole body. At one time seeking fresh air was just a matter of being out of the house. Unfortunately in these polluted times we have to look actively for places where the air is fit to breathe. Make plans to be in the countryside or by the sea as much as possible, and during the week spend your lunch break in any green space, away from cars, that you can find; trees help to absorb pollution.

Electrical pollution

Emissions of smoke and fumes from industry and motor vehicles are well known to foul the air and most people avoid such polluted areas when they can. Less well known is the effect on human health of electrical pollution. Living or working near high-voltage electricity cables has been clearly shown to affect the immune system and cause depression. We also live and work in electrically polluted spaces – badly ventilated rooms filled with electrical equipment such as VDUs, television sets, electric fires, cookers and fridge freezers. While you cannot avoid having these items around you, you can be more aware of their effects and take some simple precautions to make your environment safer: keeping rooms well ventilated, not sitting too near the television set, taking frequent breaks from your VDU set and fitting a screen protector (from Cirrus Associates – see Useful addresses).

Electrical pollution can be harmful to the body both because of the production of positive ions and also by the effect on the bio-electrical system.

Many people get headaches when there are changes in barometric pressure during hot, windy weather or during the full phase of the moon. Part of the problem is a high concentration of positive ions in the air. More about this follows.

Ions

At the end of last century scientists discovered that air electricity comes from molecules or ions of gas; each molecule has a positively charged core of protons and neutrons surrounded by negatively charged electrons. In stable air there should be equal amounts so that they cancel each other out. In electrically unbalanced air, the electron, which is lighter, is displaced and an ion is created. So unbalanced air is made of molecules that have either lost or attracted a negative electron. If a molecule loses an electron it becomes positively charged. If the displaced electron attaches to a normal molecule, that molecule becomes negatively charged. The energy that disturbs normal air and creates charged molecules is radiation.

In nature tiny amounts of radioactive substances come from the earth and the rays of the sun. Nature balances air at about five positive to four negative ions; 1000–2000 ions per cubic centimetre of air are necessary for healthy life. Scientific tests have proved that at levels significantly lower than this, plants and animals do not survive (Soyka, 1978).

Without ions we could not absorb oxygen in the quantities we need to function and it has been clearly demonstrated that the nervous system is calmer, sleeping is better and people are more cheerful where the concentration of negative ions is high.

Disturbances of the normal electrical charge of the air

Hot winds, thundery conditions and electrical equipment can all overload the air with positive ions. When the moon is full, because a positively charged layer of air is pushed nearer to the earth, the number of positive ions increases. Air high in positive ions raises serotonin levels in the brain. Serotonin is an important neuro-hormone and its part in headaches and migraines has already been discussed. Overproduction of serotonin produces hyperactivity, followed by exhaustion, anxiety and depression. The increase in serotonin levels in weather-sensitive people can cause the 'serotonin irritation syndrome': migraine, hot flushes, irritability ('lunar madness'), sleeplessness, breathing problems, tension, anxiety, digestive problems, dry husky throats, itchy noses, swollen mucosa and conjunctivitis. Breathing air high in positive ions stimulates hista-mine production, which triggers allergies. This often leads people to believe the pollen count is high when in fact their problems are caused by air high in positive ions.

Negative ions

Negative ions reduce the amount of serotonin in the brain. Concentrations of negative ions are high in the country, particularly by running water, in mountainous areas, by the sea and even in the shower. Pollutants such as smoke destroy them immediately.

Ionizers

These are machines which generate negative ions and clean the air. Domestic models are about the size of a small radio. There are smaller ones which fit into a car and much larger ones for industrial usage. Inside the plastic case a negative voltage is applied to sharp needles, causing a high-energy reaction to occur at the tip so that electrons are shot off at high velocity and collide with air molecules to form negative ions. These emerge from the ionizer in a stream. This stream, the 'ion wind', can be felt against the skin as a slight cool breeze. They are available in the electrical department of most good department stores or by mail order from health magazines. When positioning your ionizer make sure the air can circulate freely around it. Keep it away from the wall because the dust it extracts can cause discoloration; you might want to place a sheet of paper or cloth behind the ionizer on the stand to collect falling dust. Do not worry about this dust – it it better on the table than in your lungs.

Daylight – essential for health

When looking at ways to improve the general health, the effect of daylight on the body is greatly underestimated. This is not only because changes in lifestyle have deprived a large proportion of the population of exposure to daylight but also because many people who are keen to get fit spend their time in indoor leisure complexes, weightlifting, doing aerobics and so on.

In the last decade, the effect of light on human health has been the subject of increasing scientific inquiry. Biologists have discovered that not only is it vital for our well-being, but also that individual requirements for light vary as much as individual needs for vitamins. As man has become more civilized he has spent less time outdoors, and many people travel to work by car to badly lighted buildings and then return home by car to spend an evening indoors watching television. Light deprivation in humans is not as obvious as in plants, which would wilt if placed in a dark corner, or as in some animals, which are full of energy at dawn and sleep at twilight, but there is no doubt that spending too much time indoors – and also the reduced light of the shorter days of autumn and winter – do adversely affect some people.

How does light affect the body?

Daylight is necessary for normal brain functioning and for the regulation of the sleep–wake cycle. When daylight enters the eye it stimulates the pineal gland and inhibits the production of a substance called melatonin; normally this is only produced at night in the dark.

(For information on melatonin supplementation contact New Nutrition – see Useful addresses.) This is what makes us sleep. It also aids digestion and helps the production of vitamin D, and this, in turn, aids the absorption of calcium, phosphorus and magnesium.

What happens when we are starved of light

There is loss of concentration, the immune system becomes depleted and we feel lethargic, anxious and depressed. An extreme form of this is what is known as 'winter blues' or seasonal affective disorder (SAD). When the days shorten in autumn, sufferers experience symptoms which grow worse during winter, and they can be profoundly depressed. They also experience lethargy, loss of interest in sex, have joint pains and digestive problems, crave sweet foods and lack concentration to such a degree that they cannot continue their work or studies. They have great difficulty getting out of bed in the mornings and are exhausted all day. Their lack of concentration may be so severe that they have to abandon their studies or give up work. As spring approaches the symptoms abate and usually by May sufferers feel well, but are often very frustrated by the disruption in their lives and by the knowledge that they will have the same to face the following winter.

Fortunately, it has been found that being exposed, for several hours daily, to light which replicates daylight (full-spectrum light), cures this condition. This approach is now being used in hospitals in preference to drug-based therapy; even better news is that these lights are now available for large areas such as offices or therapy areas and also as small transportable units which can stand on a table for use in the home.

Benefits in the office – reduction in absenteeism and improved productivity

- Boosting of immune system reduces incidence of colds and flu.
- Helps to avoid onset of heart disease by dilating arteries and strengthening heart action.
- Helps depression by stimulating endocrine system and circulation.
- Helps fatigue by improving glucose metabolism and increasing blood flow to brain and muscles.
- Increased blood flow to brain helps concentration.
- Provides clearer illumination with high levels of definition and therefore reduces eye strain.

Benefits in the therapy room

Simultaneous benefit to patient and therapist: when a unit was fitted in the Spar Clinic at Tring, workers were better able to maintain energy throughout the day and the incidence of coughs and colds decreased.

Benefits in the home

The unit can be used by the whole family. It is safe and no special goggles are needed. It is normally used for half an hour or one hour daily, but can also be used as background lighting. Weary housewives can relax in front of it when the children have gone to school, tired husbands can come home to it and students can do their homework in front of it.

The results with ME patients who use full-spectrum light daily are very encouraging.

To understand more about the importance of daylight see Downing, 1988. For information on full-spectrum lighting contact Spectra Lighting Limited (see Useful addresses).

Sunlight

While it is foolish to risk skin cancer or ageing the skin prematurely from baking in the sun for hours, it is equally foolish never to allow the air and sun to reach the body. Frequent exposure for short periods has many beneficial effects, including the production of vitamin D. We look healthier after a little sun and this increases feelings of well-being. Sunlight also kills bacteria and fungus.

The sun headache

This is a headache caused by the sun beating down on the top of the head; it is not caused by flickering sunlight, which can trigger migraine. You can avoid both types by wearing a hat and sunglasses.

Useful addresses

Abbey Brook Cactus Nursery
Dept CP
Bakewell Road
Matlock
Derbyshire DE4 2QJ

Sells the cactus *Cereus peruvianus*, which has been shown to absorb electromagnetic radiation from VDUs and televisions.

Action Against Allergy
Amelia Hill
43 The Downs
London SW20 8HG

AAA (Action Against Allergy) provides an information service on all aspects of allergy and allergy-related illness, free to everyone. Supporting members get a newsletter three times a year and a postal lending-library service. AAA can supply GPs with the names and addresses of specialist allergy doctors. It also has a talkline network which puts sufferers in telephone touch with others through the NHS and self initiates and supports research. Please enclose s.a.e. (9 × 6 in) for further information.

Angelic Advice
3 Hutton Terrace
Sandyford
Newcastle upon Tyne NE2 1QT
Tel: 0411 010562

Bowtech
38 Portway
Frome
Somerset BA11 1QU
Tel: 01373 461 873

Contact for details of nearest therapist of or training in Bowen Therapy – a simple touch therapy for chronic pain, which is becoming inceasingly popular.

BioCare Ltd
54 Northfield Road
Norton
Birmingham B30 1JH
Tel: 0121 433 3727

Wide range of nutritional supplements for candida control and allergies including: Mycropryl (slow-release caprylic acid), Cystoplex (cranberry juice capsules), butyric acid complex (food allergies). Biocare is the only UK company in the practitioner market that manufactures its own range of Probiotics – live bacterial supplements to kill off harmful organisms in the gut – in its own facilities. BioCare's Bio-Acidophilus is the only Probiotic in the UK market derived from a research grant from the British Department of Trade and Industry.

British Holistic Medical Association
179 Gloucester Place
London NW1 6DX

British Migraine Association
178a High Road
Byfleet
Weybridge
Surrey KT14 7ED

British Society for Nutritional Medicine
PO Box 3AP
London W1A 3AP

Write for nearest doctor trained in nutritional medicine. You might need a referral letter from your GP.

Cirrus Associates
Food and Environmental Consultancy
Little Hintock
Kington Magna
Gillingham
Dorset SP8 5EW
Tel: 01747 838165

A wide range of products including VDU screen protectors, allergy-safe kettles and cooking appliances. Advice on allergies and special diets.

Colonic International Association
16 Drummond Ride
Tring
Herts HP23 5DE
Tel: 01442 827687

Family Health & Nutrition
PO Box 38
Crowborough
Sussex TN6 2YP

Federation of Aromatherapists
46 Dalkeith Road
London SE21 8LS

Ivan Frazer
49 Trevor Terrace
North Shields
Tyne & Wear NE30 2DF
Tel: 0191 290 1265

Looking for spiritual truths, uncovering suppressed esoteric, medical, scientific and political information. Quarterly magazine: *The Truth Campaign* (subscription £10).

Health Plus Ltd
PO Box 86
Seaford
East Sussex BN25 4ZW
Tel: 01323 492096

Suppliers of convenient candida control pack, Cantrol, and other products.

Herbs of Grace
Peter Enkel
5 Turnpike Road
Red Lodge
Bury St Edmunds
Suffolk IP28 8JZ
Tel: 01638 750140

Counselling on and supply of herbal remedies for migraine and other health problems.

Higher Nature
Burwash Common
East Sussex TN19 7LX
Mail order – Tel: 01435 882880; Fax: 01435 883720
Team of qualified nutritionists available to give advice –
Tel: 01435 883964

Higher Nature is dedicated to providing a comprehensive nutritional service. The quality of supplements is excellent and their Nutrition and Beyond offprints are well worth 20p. Higher Nature makes regular contributions of supplements and money to refugees and those in nutritional need. They also have an outstanding range of skin care products (Annemarie Borlind).

Hyperactive Children's Support Group
59 Meadowside
Angmering
Littlehampton
West Sussex BN16 4BW

Institute of Allergy Therapists
Short courses in the diagnosis and treatment of allergic conditions. The institute maintains a register of practitioners and provides a referral service for the general public. Write to: Donald M. Harrison, BA (Hons), BSc, MR Pharm S, Institute of Allergy Therapists, Ffynnonwen, Llangwyryfon, Aberystwyth, Dyfed SY23 4EY.

Life Tools
Department SC 1
Sunrise House
Hulley Road
Macclesfield
Cheshire SK10 2LP

Suppliers of compact machine (Mind Lab) which works with light and sound frequencies (light frames and earphones) to alter brain wave patterns to promote relaxation and sleep, or raise energy and concentration levels. Can be extremely effective for tension head-aches. Some migraine sufferers have found it beneficial after continued use. Initially there may be an increase in symptoms. Contraindicated with epilepsy.

Available for 15-day trial (UK), longer overseas. (Comes with plug adaptor for country of use.)

Lifeline Natural Foods
Mail Order Service
42 Princes Street
Yeovil
Somerset BS20 1EQ

Medical Devices Instrumentation Ltd
Cobbs Yard
St Nicholas Street
Diss
Norfolk IP22 3LB

Maker of Empulse, a simple battery operated device, worn on the body. It has greatly helped many migraine sufferers. Details available of nearest practitioner (usually a doctor or an osteopath).

Migraine Trust
45 Great Ormond Street
London WC1N 3HD
Tel: 0171 278 2676

National Institute of Medical Herbalists
41 Hatherley Road
Winchester
Hants SO22 6RR

National Society for Research into Allergy
PO Box 45
Hinckley
Leicestershire LE10 1JY

Neurolinguistic Programming is a relatively new form of counselling (sometimes available on the NHS) which often produces very rapid results with all stress-related problems:

Keith Stead
75 Townsend Crescent
Kirkhill
Morpeth NE61 2XT
Tel: 0191 268 0892

Gary Lintern
Northern College of Hypnosis
10 Thornfield Gardens
Ashbrook
Sunderland
Tyne & Wear SR2 7LD
Tel: 0191 514 4100

Vicki Whelan
Clinical Hypnotherapist, NLP (NHS & Dentistry)
The Gatehouse
Ashton Lane
Sale
Cheshire M33 6WQ
Tel: 0161 976 2716

For a therapist in your area, contact:

PO Box 48
Stourbridge
West Midlands
DY8 4ZJ
Tel: 01384 443939

New Nutrition
Penny Davenport
Woodlands
London Road
Battle
East Sussex TN33 0LP
Tel: 01424 774103

Nutritional advice for all health problems; Health Letter service; telephone and personal consultations; send s.a.e. for details.

Nutrition Associates
Galtres House
Lysander Close
Clifton Moorgate
York YO3 0XB
Tel: 01904 691591

Medical practice: candida/allergy testing, nutritional profiles, full-spectrum lighting.

Nutrition Line, see New Nutrition

The Nutritional Partnership – Individual programmes to treat the root causes of your health problems:

The Society for the Promotion of Nutritional Therapy
PO Box 47
Heathfield
East Sussex TN21 8ZX

Send £1 plus s.a.e. for a list of nutritional therapists in your area.

The Patients' Association
Room 33
18 Charing Cross Road
London WC2 0HR
Tel: 0171 240 0671

Pre-Menstrual Tension Advisory Service
PO Box 268
Hove
East Sussex BN3 1RW

Counselling for candida and cystitis; also books and videos: phone
Angela Kilmartin 0171 249 8664

Professional Association of Alexander Teachers
c/o Ian Whaley
14 Kingsland
Newcastle upon Tyne
NE2 3AL
Tel: 0191 281 8032

Sanford Clinic
15 Lake Road North
Roath Park
Cardiff CF2 5QA
Tel: 01222 747507

Society for Environmental Therapy
3 Atherton Street
Ipswich
Suffolk IP4 2LD

Society of Homoeopaths
2 Artizan Road
Northampton
NN1 4HU
Tel: 01604 21400

Spectra Lighting Limited
York House
Harlestone
Northampton NN7 4EW
Tel: 01604 821904
Fax: 01604 821902

Spiritual Counselling (Energy Medicine): Ray Abraham is a spiritual
healer and teacher who has developed a unique technique for
balancing body energies. For appointments phone 01626 853783.

Keith Thompson
20a Derwent Street
Sunderland SR1 3NU
Tel: 0191 510 1322 (phone for details on postal readings)

Provides health readings by post from garment label worn by
sufferer – electromagnetic field (auric). Helps doctors with
diagnosis.

Thursday Plantation
Illingworths
York House
York Street
Bradford BD8 0HR
Tel: 01274 488511

Hazel White-Cooper and R. S. Hom
18 Wilmington Close
Tudor Grange
Kenton Bank Foot
Newcastle upon Tyne NE3 2SF

Wholefood (organically grown produce)
24 Paddington Street
London W1M 4DR

Dr Andrew Wright
The Complete Hormone Clinic
57 Chorley New Road
Bolton
Lancs BL1 4QR
Tel: 01204 366101

Further reading

Alun-Jones, V. A., et al., 1982, 'Food intolerance: a major factor in the pathogenesis of irritable bowel syndrome', *Lancet*, 2, pp. 1115–17.

Antony, M., 1971, 'Histamines and serotonin in cluster headaches', *Archives of Neurology*, 25 (11 September), pp. 225–31.

Ashton, C. H., 1987, 'Caffeine and health', *British Medical Journal*, 295 (6609), p. 1293

Berger, B. G., and Owen, D. R., 1983, 'Mood alteration with swimming', *Psychosomatic Medicine*, 45, pp. 425–33.

Blau, J. N., 1991, *Understanding Headaches and Migraine*, Which? Books.

British Medical Journal, 1968 (14 December).

British National Formulary, 1994, 27 (March).

Brostoff, J., and Gamlin, L., 1989, *The Complete Guide to Food Allergy and Intolerance*, Bloomsbury.

Budd, Martin, 1981, *Low Blood Sugar (Hypoglycaemia): The Twentieth-Century Epidemic?*, Thorsons.

Couturier, E. G., 1993, 'The smart person will never sleep late: "weekend headache" due to late and insufficient intake of caffeine', *Ned Tijdschr Genceskd*, 137 (39: 25 September)

Davies, Stephen, 1983, 'Magnesium in health, disease and practice', *Journal of Alternative Medicine*, (December), p. 17.

Davies, Stephen, and Stewart, Alan, 1987, *Nutritional Medicine*, Pan Books.

Diamond, Harvey and Marilyn, 1987, *Fit for Life*, Bantam.

Dick, Russell, 1990, *The Temporomandibular Joint*, available from The Croft, Durham Road, Birtley, Chester-le-Street, Durham DH3 1LY.

Downing, Dr Damien, 1988, *Daylight Robbery: The Importance of Sunlight to Health*, Arrow.

Freedman, B. J., 1977, 'A diet free from additives in the management of allergic disease', *Clinical Allergy*, 7, pp. 417–21.

Gelb, Harold, 1983, *Killing Pain without Prescription*, Thorsons.

Graham, Judy, 1984, *Evening Primrose Oil: Its Remarkable Properties and Its Use in the Treatment of a Wide Range of Conditions*, Thorsons.

Grant, Ellen, 1985, *The Bitter Pill – How Safe is the 'Perfect Contraceptive'?*, Elm Tree Books.

Greden, J. F., Victor, B. S., Fontains, P., and Lubetsky, M., 1980, 'Caffeine-withdrawal headache: a clinical profile', *Psychosomatics* 21 (5).

Henderikus, J. S., McGrath, P. A., and Brooke, R. I., 1984, 'The treatment of the temporomandibular joint syndrome through control of anxiety', *Journal of Behavioural Therapeutics and Experimental Psychiatry*, 15 (1), pp. 41–5.

Horrobin, D. F., ed., 1982, *Clinical Uses of Essential Fatty Acids*, Eden Press.

Hyman, Engelberg, 1992, 'Low-serum cholesterol and suicide', *Lancet*, 339 (21 March), p. 727.

Jenkins, H. R., et al., 1984, 'Food allergy: the major cause of infantile colitis', *Annals of Allergy*, 153 (October).

Katahan, M., 1986, *The Food Rotation Diet*, Bantam.

Kripke, D. F., 1985, 'Therapeutic effects of light in depressed patients', *Annals of the New York Academy of Science*, 435.

Kushi, Mishio, 1985, *Diabetes and Hypoglycaemia: A Natural Approach*, Japan Publications.

Kuvaeva, I., et al., 1984, 'Microecology of the gastrointestinal tract and the immunological status under food allergy', *Nahrung* 28 (6–7), pp. 689–93.

Larson, Eric W., 1993, 'Migraine with typical aura associated with fluoxetine therapy', *Journal of Clinical Psychiatry*, 54 (6).

Lumb, L. C., 1981, 'Hyperventilation and anxiety state', syndromes in medicine and psychiatry: a review', *Journal of the Royal Society of Medicine*, 74 (January).

Lumb, L. C., 1987, 'Hyperventilation syndromes in medicine and psychiatry: a review', *Journal of the Royal Society of Medicine*, 80 (April).

Mackarness, Dr Richard, 1977, *Not All in the Mind*, Pan Books.

Mackarness, Dr Richard, 1985, *A Little of What You Fancy*, Fontana.

Magrath, Amy, *One Man's Poison – The 'Glucose' Factor*, available from Cirrus Associates (see Useful addresses). A mother's struggle to identify the glucose factor in carbohydrate, turning her children from unhealthy 'devils' to healthy 'angels'.

Morgan, W. P., 1979, 'Anxiety reduction following acute physical activity', *Psychiatry Annals*, 9, pp. 141–7.

Morse, D. R., 1984, 'Stress and bruxism', *Journal of Human Stress*, 8, pp. 43–54.

Mumby, Keith, 1985, *The Food Allergy Plan*, Unwin.

Neesby, Toren, 1990, 'Butyric acid complexes – a new approach to food intolerances', *Biomed Newsletter*, 1 (2).

North East Times, 1989.

O'Keefe, S. J. D., and Marks, V., 1977, 'Lunchtime gin and tonic as a cause of reactive hypoglycaemia', *Lancet*, 1, p. 1286.

Paterson, Barbara, 1985, *The Allergy Connection*, Thorsons.

Register, O., et al., 1972, *Journal of the American Dietetics Association*, 61, pp. 159–62.

Rothera, Ellen, 1988, *Perhaps It's an Allergy*, Food & Chemical Allergy Association.

Sachs, Alan, 1994, *Beyond Nutrition* (Winter).

Sachs, Oliver, 1970, *Migraine: Understanding a Common Disorder*, Faber and Faber.

San Jose Mercury News, 1993, 'A diet for drunken drivers', 7 December.

Saper, Joel R., and Magee, Kenneth R., 1978, *Freedom from Headaches*, Consumers Union of United States Inc.

Soyka, Fred, 1978, *The Ion Effect*, Bantam.

Taylor, Ron, 1986, 'Drugs and glucose tolerance', *Adverse Drug Reaction Bulletin* (Newcastle Health Authority), 121 (December)

Trickett, Shirley, 1989, *Coping with Anxiety and Depression*, Sheldon Press.

Trickett, Shirley, 1990, *The Irritable Bowel Syndrome and Diverticulosis*, Thorsons.

Trickett, Shirley, 1992, *Coping Successfully with Panic Attacks*, Sheldon Press.

Trickett, Shirley, 1994, *Coping with Candida*, Sheldon Press.

Trickett, Shirley, 1995, *Recipes for Health: Candida Albicans*, Thorsons. Although the recipes in this book are designed to discourage fungal overgrowth in the bowel, since they are sugar-free and low in carbohydrate they are equally useful for controlling low blood sugar problems. They are designed to fit in with family meals.

Trickett, Shirley, 1998, *Coming off Tranquillisers and Sleeping Pills*, 3rd ed., Thorsons.

Trimmer, Eric, 1987, *The Magic of Magnesium*, Thorsons.

Walker, J., et al., 1993, 'Analgesic rebound headache: experience in a community hospital', *Southern Medical Journal*, 86 (11), pp. 1202–5.

Werbach, Melvyn R., 1987, *Nutritional Influences on Illness: A Sourcebook of Clinical Research*, Thorsons.

Wright, Celia, 1986, *The Wright Diet*, Grafton.

Young, Sophie, 1993, 'Pilot study concerning the effects of extremely low frequency electromagnetic energy on migraine', *Journal of Alternative and Complementary Medicine* (October).

Index